HOMOE
FOR PREGNANCY AND
NURSING MOTHERS

Julie
Bagnall
1998

By the same author:-

Homoeopathic Medicine

The Homoeopathic Treatment of Emotional Illness

A Woman's Guide to Homoeopathy

Understanding Homoeopathy

Talking About Homoeopathy

An Encyclopedia of Homoeopathy

The Principles, Art and Practice of Homoeopathy

Emotional Health

Personal Growth and Creativity

The Side-Effects Book

HOMOEOPATHY FOR PREGNANCY AND NURSING MOTHERS

A Guide to Remedies for the Future Family

by

Dr Trevor Smith
MA, MB, BChir, DPM, MFHom

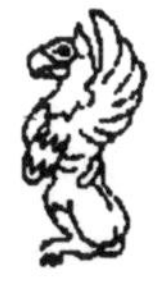

INSIGHT
Insight Editions
Worthing, Sussex
England

WARNING

The contents of this volume are for general interest only and individual persons should always consult their medical adviser about a particular problem or before stopping or changing an existing treatment.

Insight Editions
Worthing
Sussex
England

Published by Insight Editions 1993

British Library Cataloguing in Publication Data

A catalogue record for this book is available from the British Library.

ISBN 0 496670 17 X

Cover photograph by the author.

INTRODUCTION

Homoeopathy is a safe natural way of treating your baby or young child, using diluted natural extracts of plant or mineral origin. These provide a safe gentle stimulus to health.

Homoeopathy deals with the whole person, but what is most important, it deals with the psychological needs of the individual child.

Its guiding principle is treating 'like by like' - choosing a remedy which in its original form was capable of producing symptoms similar to those the child may be experiencing in his illness.

Homoeopathy supports the young mother who wants more initiative and to be more involved in the care of the family. It provides an independent approach to health problems, ensuring a safe method which supports the subtle energies of the child, responsible for its resistance and health.

Once the homoeopathic approach is understood, the mother can approach the problem with confidence, which reassures the child.

Although most mothers have heard about homoeopathy, they are not always well informed by the health visitor or midwife about its value. It is understandable therefore, that she tends to be sceptical and cautious. Being a mother can be worrying, and many mothers feel in a dilemma, trapped by the wish to use a natural method, but fearing disapproval from their General Practitioner, if he does not support homoeopathy.

Most mothers are concerned about the long-term health effects of repeated prescriptions for drugs, antibiotics, ointments or creams, upon a child.

Homoeopathy offers a safe alternative for many illnesses without side-effects. When a conventional remedy is needed for the child's health, homoeopathic remedies support the action of a drug, without reducing its activity, neutralising its action, or causing any form of adverse interaction.

It is perfectly safe to give the child a homoeopathic remedy together with a conventional drug (such as an antibiotic), as long as it is given as follows:-

Homoeopathic remedies should always be taken on a clean mouth, at least half-an-hour away from food or drink, other than water, and all other drugs or remedies.

Every young mother can get into a panic when her crying baby has wind or colic, and demands instant relief from discomfort. But try to keep a sense of calm, fun, and balance with your child at all times. Enjoy playing, and talk, hold and touch him.

If you find your child difficult at times, remember that being difficult is often a sign of intelligence and frustration at being unable to express himself.

7 Upper Harley Street
London NWI 4PS

ADVICE ON TAKING HOMOEOPATHIC REMEDIES

The remedies recommended throughout the book should be purchased directly from a homoeopathic pharmacy or health shop. Always ensure that your remedies are purchased in the 6c potency and from a reliable source.

The potencies or strengths, come as small round pills or tablets, made of sucrose (or lactose). If you are sensitive to lactose, you should order your remedies directly from a homoeopathic pharmacy, requesting a sucrose or lactose-free pill base for the remedies.

Because the medicine or homoeopathic dilution is applied directly to the surface of the pill, they should not be handled. They are best placed directly into the mouth from the lid of the container, and sucked under the tongue. They should always be taken at least 30 minutes before or after food or drink (except water); orthodox medicines; vitamin or mineral supplements; and toothpaste.

Do not drink peppermint tea when taking homoeopathic remedies. Avoid coffee, tea, and cocoa, because their high caffeine content may diminish the homoeopathic effect.

The medicines should be stored in a cool, dry, dark area, away from strong odours, especially camphor, oil of wintergreen, perfume, essential oils, after-shave, and soap. In this way, their action will last indefinitely.

A bland diet is recommended, not eating to excess, or using strong spices. Alcohol should be avoided, and smoking should be reduced or stopped altogether during the period of treatment, especially if the patient is suffering from a lung, heart, or circulatory problem.

Remedies should be taken for as long as any symptoms persist - and then stopped. If new symptoms arise during homoeopathic treatment, they should be watched carefully, especially if they have occurred in the past. The homoeopathic action may sometimes cause earlier symptoms to reappear. These are usually fleeting, but if persistent, they will require a new remedy.

An aggravation of symptoms, after taking the remedies, is a positive sign. It is usually short-lived, and does not undermine the overall sense of well-being. Do not continue taking a remedy once the symptoms have improved.

There are no side-effects or risks from homoeopathy. If you take a wrong remedy, or a whole box of the 6c pills, they will cause no harm. The remedies can be safely used during pregnancy, breast-feeding, or given to the youngest baby.

Homoeopathic remedies do not interact with orthodox medicines, or undermine their action. If you are given a course of antibiotics, it is best to stop all homoeopathic remedies until the course of antibiotics has been completed. Some orthodox drugs, especially steroids, may reduce or neutralise the homoeopathic effect.

Homoeopathy is not a treatment for acute or severe pain, and orthodox treatment is recommended if this occurs. Homoeopathy acts at every age, the reaction varying with age, strength, and the resistance or vital energy reserves of the patient. It acts very quickly in a child, or fit young person, but is slower in an elderly person, particularly if old, weak, or feeble.

It is often better initially, to give an orthodox treatment to an elderly person during the acute stage of an illness, using homoeopathy when they are recovering, or before they are in acute illness or weakness.

Homoeopathy is nevertheless helpful in the older age group, especially for stiffness, constipation, insomnia or anxiety. It does not cause confusion or agitation, which may be a severe problem when orthodox drugs are used.

BREAST ABSCESS

This sometimes occurs following a sore or cracked nipple, but it is now a fairly rare condition. It is very painful, with inflammation of the breast tissue. The breast is hard, sensitive and it may be red. The temperature is often raised, with tender lymph nodes in the axilla or armpit.

Depending on the position and degree of tenderness of the abscess, it may not be possible to breast feed with the affected breast until the condition has improved, but it should be possible to express the milk, using a breast-pump.

The baby should be given the unaffected breast, maintaining stimulation, until the condition subsides. Supplements may be necessary for a short period.

Antibiotics are usually given in conventional treatment, but they also affect the baby because they pass through the breast barrier. For this reason homoeopathy is highly recommended and without risk for the mother or child. The condition must however always be treated under medical care. Surgical drainage of the area may be required when there is pus formation.

Remedies to consider:

Belladonna	The whole affected breast feels heavy, throbbing and painful. It is hard, the skin bright red. Any sudden jolting movements increases the pain, also when lying down.
Bryonia	The breast is hot and very painful, the pain aggravated by movement or heat.
Mercurius	The breast is very painful, raw and tender, the pain worse at night in bed and for any change of temperature.
Phytolacca	There is a severe breast abscess, the area looks purple from the acute inflammation, aggravated by cold or damp conditions.
Silicea	A remedy for the more run-down, thin and exhausted mother who is plagued by recurrent infections which form a boil or abscess and discharge pus.

ALCOHOL

Most mothers naturally restrict alcohol intake during their pregnancy sensing the potential risks for them and their baby. Even occasional social drinking is best kept strictly minimal throughout pregnancy and preferably avoided altogether until breast-feeding has ended. The least alcohol amount of intake entails a definite risk for the developing foetus, depending upon amounts taken and how frequently.

The babies of mothers who drink during pregnancy tend to be underweight, more irritable and restless with difficulties in sustaining a sleep pattern and behaviour problems. The head is smaller, the face sometimes flattened. Alcohol-related heart abnormalities may occur. In severe cases of maternal alcoholism, the baby may be born with mental subnormality.

Alcohol is best avoided totally in pregnancy because it is difficult to know exactly how much is safe for the mother to take without harming the foetus. Even quite small daily amounts, two glasses of wine or two pints of beer, may be sufficient to cause harm, although some mothers are able to drink much more without harming their baby. There is also a risk that because of gastritis from the alcohol intake, the mother develops a vitamin B deficiency, which effects foetal growth.

Where the couple regularly take large amounts of alcohol, this tends to adversely effect their physical and psychological health, causing tension and anxiety, which eventually undermines the future health of the couple and their baby.

Remedies to consider:

Avena sat	A useful remedy for mild problems of this kind.
Natrum mur	This is indicated where there is severe underlying lack of confidence and depression.
Nux vomica	A remedy to consider for quite severe alcoholic problems of pregnancy, associated with sudden spasms of mood change, and irritability.
Silicea	To be considered for the thin, anxious, tense and fearful, exhausted mother lacking confidence and drive.
Sulphur	A remedy to consider for chronic problems, the mother usually overweight, intolerant of heat in any form and often vague and unsure of her directions and future. Diarrhoea with gassy indigestion is also usually present. The appetite is often insatiable.

AMBIVALENT FEELINGS

At the end of the pregnancy, when the baby is settled to the breast or bottle, the mother can relax a little more, although she is usually tired for several weeks, sometimes aggravated by the baby waking for a night-time feed or if colicky and crying at night.

Psychologically there are profound emotional changes and the woman has to change her role from pregnancy into that of the caring nurturing mother to an often very demanding baby. At this time the mother feels a variety of shifting 'peculiar'feelings, which may seem totally out of keeping with her usual self. Often she experiences feelings of being infantile herself, wanting to be held and cuddled, as well as more adult needs to be valued, reassured, and understood. She particularly wants her emotional mood swings, joy, laughter, frustration and rage, the 'blues', to be accepted by her partner, and discussed in an open way.

Many women feel some ambivalent feelings, at the end of a tiring confinement, often because they are mildly depressed, especially in the evening when tired. It is quite normal to feel some mixed feeling towards your husband or the baby, because of the psychological and hormonal changes which occur after the delivery. The best approach is to discuss them with your partner, and if they are in any way overwhelming, they should be discussed with either your doctor or health visitor.
Try to rest and to sleep as much as possible. Ignore the housework. Aim to get out of the house for some part of the day and discuss your feelings with friends without feeling guilty. Avoid isolation and negative feelings which you do not discuss with anyone close.

Remedies to consider;

China	A remedy to consider where apathy and exhaustion are major problems, also recurrent bouts of an elevated temperature. All symptoms are worse for draughts of air and cold.
Natrum mur	There is a severe loss of all confidence and drive, often with underlying depression. Tearfulness and withdrawal from others is characteristic.
Nux vomica	A very useful remedy when there is a combination of irritability, depression, and often chronic constipation.
Sepia	Symptoms are usually very severe when this remedy is indicated, with complete exhaustion at the end of the day, dragging down pelvic pains and extreme irritability with indifference.

ANAL ITCHING

This is not uncommon in pregnancy and may be due to excessive amounts of mucus produced in the anal area creating a mild eczema and irritation. Other causes are haemorrhoids due to varicose veins formed within the anal veins in this area, due to the weight of the foetus on the venous flow.

In some cases, itching is psychological, associated with panic or anxiety, and usually accompanied by other signs of tension, such as restlessness or a disturbed sleep pattern.

Another familiar cause is threadworm, the parasite usually passed from a child in the family with this problem.

Other common causes are allergic eczema due to hypersensitivity to soap powder, often a biological one. In others it is due to wearing man-made fibre rather than cotton briefs. Jeans which are too tight and block any flow of air is another cause of the problem.

During pregnancy, it is particularly important to avoid tight clothes which may restrict the pelvic venous circulation.

Remedies to consider:

Carbolic acid	For long-standing problems, the mother usually overweight and easily exhausted.
Psorinum	A remedy to consider where itching is worse from warmth and aggravated by chill and cold.
Pulex	Where irritability of the anal area is associated with irritability of mood and impatience.
Radium brom	A very useful remedy for this problem, often allied with piles, anxiety and depression.
Rhus tox	For anal irritability, relieved from heat and movement.
Sulphur	This remedy is of value for chronic problems, aggravated by heat and contact with water.

ANXIETY

Anxiety, sometimes combined with agitation may occur in any mother, especially during a first pregnancy, or where there is a history of previous miscarriages. Where this has occurred, it is understandable that the mother feels more anxious at that particular time in a subsequent pregnancy.

This anniversary or grief-reaction, may occur at the eleventh or twelfth week, or later in the pregnancy, depending upon the exact time of an earlier miscarriage. Other causes relate more to the management of the delivery, what will happen to other children, or how they will cope when she is in hospital.

A mother may worry about the future, the health of the baby, will it be normal, and what will happen if the child is born deformed, retarded, or hyperactive. Many of these fears have been passed to the mother from her own parents, together with their anxieties and often their distorted fears about pregnancy, which do not match reality.

If you feel anxious during your pregnancy, the best person to discuss this with is your partner. If that does not help to allay anxiety, then talk with your doctor or health visitor. Anxiety problems can usually be dealt with easily, but feelings of this type should not be bottled up, allowed to take root or to sap confidence and energy.

Remedies to consider:

Argentum nit	A valuable remedy where there is phobic anxiety, often the mother is house-bound, lacks confidence, and always feels worse for heat and stuffy conditions.
Gelsemium	For mild problems, with mood changes and lack of energy.
Lycopodium	For anticipatory anxiety, fear of the future, of others and of going out. Most symptoms are worse in the late afternoon or early evening. Flatulence with indigestion is commonly present.
Natrum mur	To be considered when there are severe underlying emotional problems, with depression, tearfulness and major anxiety difficulties associated with lack of confidence.

ASPIRIN AND ASPIRIN-CONTAINING PREPARATIONS

These should be avoided during pregnancy unless specifically prescribed by your doctor, and should not be purchased unless there is a medical reason to do so. Aspirin crosses the placental barrier during pregnancy, and for this reason constitutes a risk to the baby. It is also excreted into the breast milk and may affect the baby at this time.

The main risk to the mother is gastric irritation and allergic reactions, such as asthma, but it is especially a risk because it may bring about a haemorrhage. Aspirin products have an effect on the clotting mechanism of the body and prolong bleeding time. In this way there is a greater risk of haemorrhage during labour, or a possibility of bleeding during the pregnancy.

During pregnancy and when breast-feeding, any Aspirin-containing pharmaceutical preparation should only be used after consultation with your doctor. At this time it is especially important to look at the labels of any over-the-counter preparation you buy for yourself. If in doubt ask the pharmacist or your doctor if it is safe.

Remedies to consider:

Salicylic acid	This remedy is specific aspirin-related problems. Dizziness with confusion is common, associated with ringing in the ears and a red and hot irritating skin.

BACKACHE

This is an increasing problem for many women as pregnancy advances, due to several factors. The weight of the growing foetus in the uterus presses upon the pelvic basin affecting the low back. Also the position of the spine changes in late pregnancy to accommodate the foetus. Back discomfort may also be caused by an increased weight gain, or from stretching of the spinal and pelvic ligaments.

It is important to keep body weight as near to the expected norm for your height and weight as possible, taking into account the stage of the pregnancy and what would be a normal weight gain at this time. If in doubt discuss this with your doctor or health visitor. Salt should be kept minimal to reduce fluid retention and also synthetic sugars should be avoided. Keep your carbohydrate intake low, especially from chocolate and pastry or cakes.

If backache is severe in late pregnancy, this is best dealt with by rest and avoidance of carrying heavy weights as from shopping or any heavy household chores. If backache occurs in early pregnancy, it is often due to a hormonal effect on the ligaments, preparing them for stretching in late pregnancy. For early pregnancy backache, exercise such as swimming and specific back-strengthening exercises are of value.

Remedies to consider:

Kali carb	A remedy for back problems with tearing pains, all symptoms worse for cold and in the early night hours, approximately 4-5.00am.
Natrum mur	This remedy is useful for chronic low back-pain, worse for cold and for firm physical pressure in the painful area.
Radium brom	There is severe pain, better for movements and heat, associated with irritability and fatigue.
Rhus tox	Useful for rheumatic back-ache, worse for cold and damp, better for heat and movement.
Ruta	This is often a useful remedy for back problems of pregnancy, especially when improved by rest, lying on a firm mattress and for firm local pressure.

BLADDER PROBLEMS

As in late pregnancy backache, the weight of the foetus and uterus tends to press down upon the bladder as the pelvic ligaments slowly become more elastic and lengthen. This tends to change slightly the position of the bladder and with it the external orifice or urethra, making it more susceptible to ascending infections.

During pregnancy it is very common for the mother to experience bladder irritability, especially frequency and at times pain and irritability, also urgency. If discomfort occurs, drink plenty of fluids and discuss the problem with your doctor.

Avoid delaying emptying the bladder for long periods which may strain the delicate bladder control mechanism.

It is important to get recurrent bladder problems treated as soon as possible. If persistent they may become chronic and lead to diminished fertility or to an ascending infection that causes kidney inflammation (pyelitis) with pain in the kidney region and a high temperature.

If you are considering a pregnancy and already have a bladder problem or weakness in this area, it is important to have it treated. Specific exercises to improve pelvic floor functioning are also recommended.

Remedies to consider:

Apis	Indicated when there are burning or scalding pains, often with small amounts of urine passed. Pain is most marked at the end of the flow.
Berberis	A remedy for more severe deep-seated problems, with burning pain on passing water, the urine often containing mucus or a sediment. All symptoms are aggravated by movement, also after standing for long periods.
Cantharis	Useful for acute inflammatory conditions with frequency and urgency. The urine feels hot and burning.
Nux vomica	A remedy for spasms of pain with irritability of mood.
Populus trem	This remedy is indicated for the most severe and painful conditions with spasm on passing water. It is often associated with severe sweating, especially at night, and a raised temperature.

BLEEDING

Loss of blood from the vagina during pregnancy is not normal and usually an indication of a threatened miscarriage. The mother should immediately rest in bed and call for medical advice. After bleeding, it is best to avoid sexual intercourse for several weeks or until the pregnancy is completely stable again.

If contractions also occur, usually felt as lower abdominal pain at the time of bleeding, this increases the likely diagnosis of a threatened miscarriage.

Complete bed rest is absolutely essential. In recurrent cases, this may be required for the remainder of the pregnancy. The most common critical times of risk are usually the eleventh or twelfth weeks and again at a later stage at twenty weeks.

In most cases the causes are unknown, but common factors are stress and hormonal failure.

If bleeding has occurred, even briefly at any time during the pregnancy, avoid excessive effort in the home or when shopping. Also avoid heavy lifting and be sensible and moderate in your approach to sport and exercising.

Remedies to consider;

Arnica	An important acute remedy for shock and whenever there is bruised lower abdominal or pelvic discomfort.
Phosphorus	Where there is a profuse loss of bright red blood with restlessness and anxiety.
Sabina	A major remedy for threatened miscarriage at twelve weeks. The loss may contain clots. Pain is usually in the low back or pelvic area. All symptoms are worse from heat and movement.
Secale	For oozing haemorrhages at the third month of pregnancy with extreme exhaustion and anxiety. All symptoms are worse for heat or when covered up and too warm.
Viburnum op	A remedy for recurrent miscarriage in the early weeks. Spasmodic pain with haemorrhage is characteristic, all symptoms worse for heat and a stuffy airless room.

BLOOD-PRESSURE

For the health of the foetus, the mother's blood-pressure should remain at normal levels throughout the pregnancy. Every mother should endeavour to keep her weight at the target level for her age, height and the stage of her pregnancy.

It is important not to put on an excessive amount of weight by eating too much carbohydrate, taking too much fluid, or additional salt, but fluids should not be restricted. A sensible dietary balance is required and regular exercise maintained throughout the pregnancy.

If the mother develops fluid retention, especially swollen ankles, or is short of breath, she should report this to her doctor or midwife. Repeated nose-bleeds, headaches, dizziness or fainting turns, should also be a signal for an immediate medical check-up.

If you do have a blood-pressure problem, try to stay as relaxed as you can throughout the pregnancy by increasing your relaxation times. Take extra rest periods, at least once a day and keep stress levels minimal.

At all times avoid getting angry or over-excited. But if you are consistently feeling uncontrollable emotions then discuss this with your doctor.

Remedies to consider:

Apis	Throbbing headaches, dizziness with fatigue are typical symptoms, the skin very sensitive to touch. Exhaustion is marked, all symptoms worse for heat and local pressure.
Digitalis	An important remedy when the pulse is slow and usually irregular, the cheeks often have a bluish tint, due to cyanosis or a lack of oxygen.
Natrum mur	This remedy is indicated for severe problems with high readings of the blood-pressure. Palpitations are a frequent problem with lack of energy.
Nux vomica	Headache, mainly across the forehead may be a problem with dizziness, indigestion problems and marked irritability.
Spigelia	A useful remedy when the major problem is a sudden racing heart beat, chest discomfort or pain, on effort, and shortness of breath.

'BLUES' AND POST-NATAL DEPRESSION

Some degree of disappointment and depression is normal after the pregnancy has ended, probably because it is an ending of a major psychological event in life and the mother may feel that she no longer has a useful role to play, or in an older woman, that she may never become pregnant again. For this reason, the birth is felt to be a loss as well as a fulfilment.

Many mothers feel tired and down for the first few weeks because they are back in the home. They may not always value their new maternal role and often feel they have lost some of their independence as if shunted into a backwater. A first-time mother often feels inadequate, unsure of herself, and feeling ashamed of having anything other than the most joyful and positive of reactions to the baby. But just after the birth is a difficult time for many women who feel unsure of themselves and just how to think about the future and wondering in what way she will act and feel different from how she was before the pregnancy started.

For many mothers, the pregnancy and arrival of the baby changes priorities as well as life-style, and sets her thinking differently, often more deeply. The experience of having the baby and giving birth, awakens quite new psychological feelings, which were not so obvious before. These may include doubts and fears about herself and the future as well as more positive strengths gained at the same time. Keep the communication doors open with your partner and don't be afraid to show need and weakness or fears. Being able to show these more vulnerable aspects of yourself always reflects a strength rather than a weakness.

Remedies to consider:-

Lycopodium	A remedy for mild depression with mainly fears of change and the future.
Pulsatilla	Recommended when the moods are changeable, accompanied by variable emotion, especially tearfulness.
Natrum mur	Of value when depression is more severe and there is loss of confidence, often with anxiety about meeting others or fear of new situations.
Nux vomica	To be considered when there is extreme irritability and short-fuse intense emotional outbursts.

AFTERPAINS

These are uterine cramps which occur a few days after birth, often as a result of breast-feeding.

Giving the breast stimulates hormonal (oxytocin) release from the pituitary area of the mid-brain, which acts directly on the uterus causing it to contract and return to its original size and position within the pelvis.

They are more common in women who have had previous deliveries.

Afterpains may appear to be a simple problem, but when combined with pain from a sore perineum and breast engorgement, they can often create severe discomfort for the mother and this is usually far worse when the mother is breast-feeding.

Remedies to consider:

Magnesium phos	A remedy to consider for very severe colicky pains, especially when right-sided and improved by warmth, firm local pressure and rest in bed.
Nux vomica	For severe spasms of lower abdominal pain, especially worse on waking and improved by damp humid conditions.

BREAST-FEEDING OR BOTTLE ?

Breast-feeding is a sensitive emotional issue. Probably it is better psychologically and physically for the health of the baby and more natural, but no mother should feel guilty if she decides not to breast-feed or if she has insufficient milk. If she feels uncomfortable about giving the breast, then she should make her own choice in the matter. She should certainly always resist pressure from the professionals to breast-feed if she doesn't feel at ease giving the breast.

The choice must rest with the individual mother, and it should not become a major psychological issue. Each mother should make her own decision. She should however try breast-feeding to see if it suits her and the baby for a few weeks.

The mother can then decide how comfortable she feels about it and if the baby is putting on sufficient weight. What matters is a reasonable choice for both mother and baby, offering what is best for the physical health of the baby and the mother, also for the bonding of mother and child.

Psychologically it is the quality of affection and closeness that is most important, how the bottle or breast is given, rather than which is chosen. Government policy is to encourage more mothers to breast-feed at birth.

In the UK, approximately 65% of mothers initiate breast-feeding. Official guidelines recommend this should rise to 75% by the year 2000, and that the present level of 40% of infants breast-fed to six weeks, should rise to 50%.

But no mother should allow her natural maternal instincts and intuition, to be imposed upon by the policy-makers. Ultimately she must decide what is best for herself and the baby without guilt, or feelings of having compromised.

If you do decide to breast-feed your baby, recent research suggests that breast milk should not be given for longer than six to nine months. A recent 1992 study, on 5,000 men, reported in the British Medical Journal and carried out in two major hospitals in the U.K., found a significantly higher death rate from heart disease and higher levels of serum cholesterol, when the male baby had been fed at the breast for a prolonged period of a year or longer.

Although breast feeding is best for your baby, if prolonged, it may have life-long repercussions on health, and some caution is needed. If in doubt, when to wean or to stop breast-feeding, always discuss this with your health visitor or doctor.

BREASTS PAINFUL

Discomfort is often felt in the breasts during pregnancy because of the speed of hormonal changes and development of the milk-producing glandular tissue, in preparation for feeding the baby.

The usual causes for problems, are these hormonal changes, resulting in fluid retention and expansion of the breast milk ducts.

The major symptoms are pain, soreness and a heavy discomfort on movement.

Most women put up with this problem without complaining, because they feel orthodox medicine has nothing to offer them and they know of no alternative approach. The condition can however be safely and effectively improved by homoeopathy.

Remedies to consider:

Belladonna	The breasts feel heavy and uncomfortable, often very hard, swollen, and burning hot. All symptoms are worse from heat, pressure or the least jarring movement.
Bryonia	There is severe stitch or tearing pains in the breasts, which are hard and feel hot. All symptoms are aggravated by heat or movement.
Pulsatilla	A remedy for mild variable breast pain, always aggravated by heat and emotion.
Sepia	There is a heavy dragging down discomfort, worse in the evening, when tired, before thunder, better for vigorous movement and exercise.

CAESARIAN SECTION

A Caesarian birth may be safest for the baby, but it may at the same time cause psychological problems for the mother, because she feels that it is not such a natural process.

The mother is not usually prepared for a Caesarian birth in her ante-natal classes, and given limited information only. Some women experience a sense of failure when the baby is born in this way. Privately she may feel cheated of the birth experience and not totally sure that the baby is really her's. This sense of doubt may sometimes cause problems in handling the baby or cause slight bonding difficulties. If the mother feels cheated, this may also cause breast feeding to fail. Post-operative pain and discomfort may also diminish lactation in some cases, because of sedation after the operation, or from a stitch abscess or suture infection.

Some post-Caesarian mothers are recommended not to drive for one month after the operation. This can lead to a mother losing confidence, becoming isolated and depressed. She may not want to be dependent, or feel a burden upon friends or relatives, preferring to stay on her own at home, rather than to go out as before.

After a Caesarian section operation, the mother should be as mobile as possible, taking gentle walks. For the first three months, to avoid excessive strain on the suture line, the mother should not carry heavy shopping or children. Extra rest from domestic chores is recommended, and the family should ensure she strictly limits the amount of physical work undertaken.

Remedies to consider:

Ignatia	A remedy when there are marked emotional features with sadness and often anxiety, the symptoms variable, and linked to a sense of loss or disappointment. All symptoms are worse for fresh air and in the morning.
Natrum mur	Useful when there is a severe emotional reaction to the birth, especially feelings of depression and lack of confidence.
Sepia	Indicated when the mother feels tired, exhausted, depressed, and very irritable to the point of indifference. All symptoms are worse in the evening and when she is tired.

COLDS AND FLU

These should be treated as soon as they appear with the appropriate homoeopathic remedies which do not pose any threat to the mother or the foetus.

If there is a high temperature, diarrhoea or vomiting, the mother may feel better if she takes fluids only until the condition has settled. If these symptoms persist, including a cough or any shortness of breath, she should consult her doctor.

Avoid cigarette smoke and smoke-filled rooms at this time, also over-heated, dry atmospheres as much as possible during pregnancy.

Contact with other flu sufferers should be avoided, or kept to a strict minimum throughout this period.

If there is a severe cold in a close member of the family, homoeopathy can also be used to prevent or limit the severity of an infection.

Remedies to consider:

Aconitum	For recent very acute febrile colds with shivering attacks, chill, restlessness and often anxiety.
Arsenicum	This is useful for an acute cold where the mother feels very chilly and particularly exhausted. All symptoms are worse after midnight.
Bryonia	A remedy for upper chest colds with a dry cough, worse for heat or movement.
Gelsemium	Indicated for mild colds with nasal congestion and a sore throat. Dizziness with fatigue and complete apathy are common.
Hepar sulph	A remedy when there is a painful throat and sinus infection, associated with a mild temperature and sharp splinter-like pains in the area affected.
Influenzinum	Useful for acute viral colds, especially during a flu epidemic.
Nux vomica	For acute colds with spasms of gastric discomfort or pain, often with constipation. Irritability of mood is marked.

CONFIDENCE

It is essential that every mother feels confident with herself and comfortable with her baby. If you are feeling anxious, then discuss this openly with your partner to try to clarify the reasons, and what may be causing them. The mother should at all times be herself, not influenced by how others seem to be, or expect her to respond. It is an error for the mother to make comparisons with other mothers, as she may devalue herself. A problem should not be turned into a failure, or treated as anything more than it is, and difficulties should not be seen as an expression of weakness. Every mother should realise that being a mother is probably the most important work and role that it is possible to have. But being a happy, relaxed, confident mother is even better. If she stays relaxed and confident, both her partner and baby benefit from the harmony and emotional balance this brings.

Each child develops his patterns of behaviour by learning from example. It is not so much what you say, but how you say it, that determines his understanding and responses. If you don't want your child to shout or swear - then don't shout or swear at the child. Don't hit the child if you don't want him to hit back at you. Try to approach all pressure situations confidently, without bribes, smacking, or physical threats. If you must punish, some form of temporary restriction is often most effective, but explain your reasons, and those aspects of his behaviour you disapprove of.
At all times, respect the child as a person and an individual, even if you feel he has behaved badly. If he has been childish and immature, this is to be expected from one only beginning to learn social behaviour.

Remedies to consider:

Kali carb	Indicated for lack of confidence, the mother also lacking energy and tending to be overweight. Most symptoms are worse in the early hours, about 4-5.00 a.m.
Natrum mur	A remedy when there are problems of insecurity and depression, the mother never feeling fully confident in any social situation and often anxious, never fully herself with others. Symptoms are either better or worse at the seaside. She is usually a loner, fearing close contact with others.
Phosphorus	For the often pale and thin mother who needs the approval of others to feel confident. She is always seeking reassurance that she is liked and acceptable.
Pulsatilla	Indicated for the shy dramatic woman with variable moods. Tearfulness and depression alternate with laughter.
Silicea	Useful where there is exhaustion, recurrent infection, with lack of resistance and body heat. Drive, determination and staying power are psychologically lacking.

CONSTIPATION

Constipation is often associated with pregnancy, and can create quite considerable lower abdominal discomfort.

Throughout the pregnancy the mother should take extra fibre as bran, and also eat foods such as prunes, fresh fruit, and baked beans, which are naturally high in fibre content.

It is important to keep fluid intake high, but avoid excessive intake of tea and coffee. Exercise regularly, but never excessively.

As far as possible, keep to a natural unprocessed diet with plenty of salads and lightly steamed vegetables a major part of each meal. Avoid laxatives and developing a dependency on them.

This is a problem where orthodox medicine has little to offer, because of the vulnerability of the young foetus. Homoeopathy is always safe and effective, giving relief to this very common problem which causes a great deal of pain anxiety and discomfort to the mother.

Remedies to consider:

Alumina This remedy is useful for severe constipation related to a high dietary intake of aluminium, either from tea or aluminium kitchen utensils. A dry skin and itchy eyes may also be present.

Bryonia There is severe constipation, aggravated by heat and worse for exercise.

Collinsonia For severe constipation with stitch-like rectal pains, often associated with haemorrhoids. All symptoms are worse from cold and improved by warmth.

Nux vomica This is a recommended for chronic constipation, often associated with spasms of gastric pain, flatulence and distention. Irritability is usually marked.

Opium Indicated for the most severe obstinate absolute constipation, often lasting for days. Drowsiness and lethargy are marked.

CONTRACEPTION

Many women wrongly believe that because they are breast-feeding and have not yet had a period, they are not ovulating and therefore there is no possibility of another pregnancy occurring.

But ovulation may occur during the time a mother is giving the breast and it is important that the couple take precautions if they do not wish for another pregnancy.

The best contraceptive method, with least risk to mother or baby, is to use a simple barrier method such as a condom with a spermicidal cream.

If the mother is breast-feeding, it will not be possible for her to return to taking the 'combined pill' (i.e. one containing oestrogen and progesterone), if this was her former method, as this combination will interfere with lactation.

The 'mini' pill (progesterone only), may be considered as an alternative. For more up-to-date information, this should be discussed with your doctor.

DISLIKE OF BREAST-FEEDING *

Most women find breast-feeding an easy natural process and a fulfilling closeness which they enjoy. It is not uncommon however for it to feel wrong from the start, and it may even seem abnormal. The mother finds it psychologically distasteful, and she may not have a 'feeling' for breast-feeding, with no desire or interest, because it seems unnatural. She does not usually mind bottle feeding, but giving her own breast just seems wrong to her.

When breast-feeding goes against these deeper instincts, it is better not to do so, nor form an unnatural relationship which does not feel right. Everyone is unique, and the mother should not feel guilty, or that she is wrong or inadequate. She should accept her own judgement, how she is and feels at the time. When she has a healthy self-relationship, she can also have a more balanced relationship to the baby, and she should not seek to force anything which seems abnormal to her, or which does not feel natural.

The underlying causes may never be known. Perhaps breast-feeding was denied to the mother, or abruptly terminated just when established because of an infection. The woman's own mother may have had problems when breast-feeding, and her negative self-imagery unconsciously transmitted to the daughter, so that she becomes too deeply identified with her. The reasons are nearly always deep-seated, and in many ways academic. What matters is that the baby is fed adequately, and thrives with closeness and affection.

* From The Side-Effects Book.

CONTRACTIONS DURING LABOUR

The strength of contractions during labour, can be helped by using homoeopathic remedies during the last three months of pregnancy, as a preparation for a natural healthy labour.

Strong, regular, contractions, help the delivery, and avoid a prolonged birth, or a possible induction of labour, which is an unnatural process.

The homoeopathic remedies mentioned support healthy uterine tone during the latter part of the pregnancy, and in this way, help prevent complications occurring.

Homoeopathy helps and supports the delivery. It also minimises the need for chemical or synthetic compounds having to be used and minimises any artificial interference.

A natural and normal delivery is ideal, giving the mother a sense of fulfilment and felt to be most satisfying psychologically.

Remedies to consider:

Caulophyllum This is a most valuable remedy to help strengthen contractions during the birth process, acting specifically on the uterine muscles and their co-ordinated action.

Cimicifuga The remedy acts on the uterus to prevent intermittent labour contractions and difficulties with labour. The remedy also helps with after-pains, and to prevent exhaustion of the uterus.

Pulsatilla A useful remedy when there are weak, variable, delayed, or false labour contractions. It is also helpful in the 3rd stage of labour, if the placenta is retained, or there are severe after-pains. There is intolerance of heat and wide mood variations, often with tears.

CRACKED NIPPLE

This is usually an extension of an untreated sore nipple problem. It is extremely painful and if left untreated may cause infection of the breast tissue (mastitis). It is **always** best treated by prevention.

If the problem is severe, a breast shield may be required for a few days, or the baby may have to be taken off the affected breast for a few days until the nipple is fully healed.

The mother is normally recommended to continue breast feeding the baby on the unaffected side. On the affected side, she is usually advised to hand-express her own milk or to use a breast-pump, giving the baby her own expressed milk rather than a supplement.

She should change breast pads regularly, and try to expose the breast to warm fresh air for half-and-hour, morning and evening, to promote healing. Small three-hourly feeds are often suggested.

Calendula cream can be usefully applied to any cracked areas to encourage healing at the same time as taking one of the homoeopathic remedies by mouth.

Remedies to consider:

Castor equi	A remedy for red, thickened irritated or cracked sore nipples. There is often a quite severe irritation of the area and they are very tender to touch or pressure.
Graphites	This is useful when the nipples are cracked and ooze a clear or straw-coloured discharge.
Nitric acid	Indicated when the nipples are very painful and tender, with sharp stitch-like pains, worse in the evening and from heat or becoming chilled.
Silicea	The nipples are cracked and infected with a thick yellow pus discharge. The mother usually feels cold and exhausted and her general vital resistance and energy is low, making her vulnerable to recurrent infections.

CYSTITIS

A bladder infection with discomfort on passing water is very common during pregnancy because of pressure from the weight of the growing foetus pressing on the bladder. This may lead to displacement or kinking of the external passage or urethra and causes infection to occur.

The usual symptoms are discomfort on passing water, often of a burning type, frequent urination and urgency, or inability to retain a full bladder. If recurrent, it may be a major cause of reduced fertility in women and inability to conceive.

During pregnancy it is very important that cystitis is treated promptly and that adequate fluids are taken. Fluid intake should not however be excessive because of the risk of overloading the circulation causing fluid retention and weight gain.

If not treated, cystitis may become chronic or a recurrent problem. In some cases the bladder infection may ascend to involve the kidneys with pyelitis. This is particularly undesirable during pregnancy.

The response to homoeopathy is usually rapid and very positive.

Remedies to consider:

Cantharis	For intense irritation with spasms of discomfort, burning pain and frequency. All the symptoms are worse on passing urine.
Formica rufa	For acute urinary irritation with an urgent need to pass urine, often associated with rheumatic pains. All symptoms are worse from cold or damp conditions.
Hepar sulph	There are stitch-like pains in the bladder area. Frequency is a common cause of discomfort.
Nux vomica	Indicated for recurrent problems, with spasms of pain, irritability, constipation, and indigestion.
Populus trem	A valuable remedy for cystitis of pregnancy with burning pain on passing water and severe spasm at the end of the flow.
Staphysagria	A remedy for painful bladder problems after delivery, particularly after an episiotomy. Spasm and ineffective urging is characteristic, often with irritable mood swings and outbursts of uncontrolled emotion.

DIET

During pregnancy a diet is required that is high in both cereal and vegetable fibre. This is present in cereals of the Muesli type which are excellent for breakfast, topped with sliced apple or banana. Fresh vegetables and fruit should be eaten daily as a salad. Eat freshly prepared meals, high in carbohydrate and protein, low in fats, but to avoid weight gain, don't eat to excess. If you are feeling hungry between meals, eat fruit or a bowl of cereal. Avoid crisps, nuts, bars of chocolate, high calorie cakes or biscuits. Whenever possible, eat organically-grown cereals, bran and vegetables to minimise intake of pesticide residues in your food.

During pregnancy there is a higher risk of contacting a listeria infection. The Listeria Monocytogenes organism has been shown to be in certain foods, and is a risk of infection or miscarriage to the pregnant mother. It is now official policy that all Camembert, Brie, and blue-veined cheeses should not be eaten during pregnancy. You should also avoid soft creamy, mouldy, and goat cheese. High levels of the listeria micro-organism have been found in other foods, especially paté, cook-chill or frozen chicken, beef, pork, lamb, crab meat, shrimps, also pre-packaged supermarket salads.

Care should be taken when using any pre-cooked frozen foods. These should be stored at the correct and recommended temperatures, away from raw foods or cheeses. They are recommended to be thoroughly re-heated until piping hot according to label instructions. If re-heating is incorrect, these foods create a high-risk source of listeria infection for the pregnant mother.

Never re-heat pre-cooked frozen foods more than once.

Most cases of Listeria Monocytogenes infection occur in pregnancy (66%) and care should be taken when the above foods are purchased. Hard and processed cheeses, cheese spread, and cottage cheese are safe to eat.

Because of the risk of Salmonella infection, pregnant women should also avoid eating raw eggs. These may be present in certain recipes, such as mayonnaise and egg custard. Eggs should be free-range and not from a battery farm, always cooked until both the white and yolk are firm. If you do want to use partially cooked eggs in a particular recipe, only use pasteurised dried or liquid egg preparations during pregnancy.

Unwashed vegetables or salads should be avoided. The pregnant mother should also avoid eating raw or partially cooked meat in any form, and she should not handle or contaminate other food with the juices of such meat. She should also wash her hands carefully after contact with raw meat, (and also after preparing pet food using raw meat, because of the risks of Toxoplasmosis. The intake of liver should be reduced or avoided (see the section on the risks of vitamin excess in pregnancy, page 147)

DRUGS

Both prescribed, and over-the-counter pharmacy preparations, should be kept strictly minimal, if possible avoided altogether during pregnancy and when breast-feeding. They should only be used under strict medical supervision, because they may place the health of the mother and the foetus at risk.

Because of the increased risk of haemorrhage, all aspirin-containing preparations should be avoided, also all iodine containing preparations, both internally, and those for local use on the skin.

All the social drugs of addiction, especially alcohol, tea, coffee, tea, cigarettes, are a high-risk factor for the foetus and should be avoided by those who regularly use them at other times.

The anti-malarial drugs may also create a risk for the vulnerable foetus and it may be advisable to delay a trip to areas where malaria is endemic until after the birth and weaning from breast-feeding. Always discuss the use of anti-malarial drugs with your doctor if you are pregnant and be fully aware of the possible risks.

DRUGS TO BE AVOIDED, OR USED WITH EXTREME CAUTION DURING PREGNANCY *

DO NOT ALTER OR STOP ANY DRUG IN PREGNANCY WITHOUT FIRST CONSULTING YOUR DOCTOR.

Analgesics (pain-relieving) remedies
Aspirin, Indomethacine, Gold compounds, Naproxen

Anti-infective remedies and antibiotics
Tetracyclines, Chloramphenicol, Antimalarial drugs

Heart and Circulation remedies
Warfarin, Ergotamine, Diuretics

Hormonal remedies
Oestrogens, Androgens, Progesterone, Stilboestrol

Intestinal remedies
Atropine, Stimulant laxatives, Sulphasalazine

Iodine preparations
Iodides, Iodine, Radioactive Iodine

Psychological remedies
Lithium, Barbiturates, Benzodiazepines, Phenothiazines

Respiratory remedies
Aminophylline, Atropine, Theophylline, Ephedrine

Vaccines
All live vaccines are dangerous

* From The Side-Effects Book

DUMMIES, DISADVANTAGES OF

The tired mother, struggling with a demanding or crying child, is tempted to give him a dummy to quieten him down. But in most cases it is not recommended for other than very minimal periods because of the damage it may do.

Every dummy is a potential source of infection and can rarely be kept either clean or sterile for more than a few minutes. It is undesirable because it creates a habit and subdues the baby who cries for a reason and not because he is naughty.

A mother should always find out the reasons why the baby is crying in order to remedy them and to reassure the baby. There are in fact very few reasons why a baby cries and every mother should quickly learn what the reasons are and be able to respond to the baby's needs without pushing a dummy into his mouth, at the same time subduing the cries of need and protest.

To always push a dummy into the baby's mouth psychologically encourages passivity and in later life, the adult may resort to similar oral (mouth) comforters - reaching for a pipe or cigarette or something sweet, sugary and reassuring - rather than admitting to a need. This is because he has been taught to do this as a child.

A dummy may also interfere and possibly in the long term, delay speech development of the young baby or child, because he needs to practice constantly his sounds and noises when at play.

Thrush is another complication of dummies and often causes the baby to have a sore mouth. As a result he may not feed happily because of pain or discomfort. He may also cry more and healthy weight gain may be affected. Persistent thrush may be transferred to the nappy area causing a sore and infected buttock region.

If the dummy is persistently given to an older child it may cause recurrent stomach or intestinal infection, particularly diarrhoea and vomiting. These problems occur more frequently in children who regularly have a dummy to pacify them than those who have not.

There is also a slight risk of a more serious accident occurring, and it has been recorded that some children have died following inhalation of the end of the dummy, which has become either detached from its base, or bitten off by the child.

The other possible risk is of dental damage to the bite. Although some modern dummies are now marketed as being less damaging to the mouth and dental development, their use should be kept minimal because of the potential risks to the child.

EAR PIERCING

Because of the possible risks of a Hepatitis type B virus infection occurring (causing inflammation of the liver), ear piercing should be avoided throughout pregnancy.

Body piercing, has now become fashionable, and all forms, including nose, umbilicus, or genital, are potentially high risk procedures and should be avoided until after the birth because of the risks of hepatitis.

For the same reason, tattoos are also not recommended during pregnancy.

Dental interventions involving the use of needles, including injections for a local anaesthetic, should also be treated with caution and if possible avoided.

Remedies to consider:

Chelidonium	A remedy with specific liver and gall-bladder action. The liver is usually enlarged and tender, or there may be colicky pains and in severe conditions, jaundice.
Phosphorus	An important treatment for liver degenerative or inflammatory disease, having the ability to help regenerate new liver growth and functioning following damage from infection, or exposure to chemicals.

ECTOPIC PREGNANCY

An ectopic pregnancy is one where fertilisation and embedding of the fertilised ovum occurs outside the uterus. The fertilised ovum may embed itself in the fallopian tube, or sometimes within the peritoneal tissues of the abdominal cavity.

In every ectopic pregnancy, there is a high risk of bleeding, pain and haemorrhage, possibly with peritonitis from bleeding into the peritoneal cavity and the risk of infection in that area.

Many ectopic pregnancies abort spontaneously at eleven or twelve weeks, sometimes later. Once diagnosed, because of severe pain and bleeding and risk to the mother, they are usually terminated surgically. There may be a higher incidence of ectopic pregnancies for those mothers who become pregnant when they are also taking the 'pill'.

Remedies to consider:

Aconitum	A remedy for shock, with exhaustion, restlessness or agitation. It is also helpful for severe shooting pains or spasm of the uterus.
Arnica	Useful for shock and collapse with pain and discomfort in the lower abdomen, the mother feels bruised as if she has been kicked in the lower pelvic area.

EPISIOTOMY - PAIN FROM

Most episiotomy (birth incision) sutures heal well and quickly. But in some cases there is pain afterwards which may last for several weeks. It is current practice to avoid an episiotomy (which is a surgical procedure), whenever possible and a small perineal tear is far preferable and heals more quickly.

The commonest cause is a stitch abscess from infection of the suture area. If this persists, it may drag the woman down psychologically and affect pelvic comfort and resumption of normal intercourse.

Bathing the area twice daily with warm salt baths is helpful. Avoid long periods of standing at household jobs which can equally be done sitting. In this way stasis (a sluggish circulation) and engorgement from the accumulation of venous blood in the area can be avoided.
Gentle walking is beneficial as long as it does not cause aggravate discomfort or pain.

Take bran daily to avoid constipation and to lessen stretching and pressure on the area from a full rectum.

Remedies to consider:

Belladonna	Useful when the pelvic area feels inflamed, red and burning hot, with dragging down pains. All symptoms are worse from touch or pressure and from jolting movements.
Calendula	A major remedy for healing episiotomy problems. It is best applied locally to the tender area as a cream, or taken internally by mouth.
Hepar Sulph	This remedy is indicated when there are sharp stitch-like pains, aggravated by touch, pressure, or cold.
Staphysagria	A valuable remedy for episiotomy pain or infection, with sharp needle-like pain, worse for pressure or sitting, with often intense irritability of mood.

EXERCISE

Daily exercise, without carrying heavy loads of shopping or a heavy handbag, is essential throughout pregnancy.

About an hour a day is sufficient, unless there is a medical reason for the mother to be completely at rest, or where exercise is contraindicated by the doctor.

Total rest without exercise may sometimes be recommended for pre-eclampsia (toxaemia of pregnancy with high blood-pressure, protein in the urine, and swollen ankles from fluid retention), or where bed rest is essential because of recurrent miscarriage.

For the majority of mothers, daily exercise is a necessity for health during the pregnancy. Walking or swimming, are ideal if available and should be continued throughout the pregnancy and when breast-feeding.

The value of exercise is primarily that it acts as a healthy stimulant to elimination, and also as a tonic to the heart, circulation, bowels and urinary functioning.

AMBIVALENT FEELINGS TO THE BABY *

Ambivalence to the new baby is common in many women during the early weeks. This also occurs in fathers, although not often openly admitted. Either parent may only be able to fully relate to the baby when it is a few weeks old and more of a little person.

Fatigue after the confinement, loss of sleep when breast-feeding, or from a baby who wakes frequently during the night, may undermine vitality and reserves, depending upon age, fitness, and also the previous emotional health of the parents.

A woman can feel trapped by her first maternal experiences, and however 'good' or healthy the baby, feel alienated from friends, routine and work. She may resent this, feeling that the man carries on as before. This can undermine the closeness of the relationship, without her being able to express 'why', often because she feels guilty. There may be less ability to express feelings of affection, need, closeness and love.

Irritability, loss of libido, exhaustion, are all common in the early weeks, and should be regarded as normal. Usually these feelings pass quickly once a feeding pattern is established. As soon as the mother-child psychological bond is secure, and also that of the father, much of the ambivalence lessens. But as with all relationships, it is always there to some extent, however close, largely replaced for most of the time, by the sense of closeness, joy and fulfilment.

* From The Side-Effects Book.

FLUID RETENTION

This is a common pregnancy problem, usually hormonal in origin, but aggravated by a high salt or sodium intake. It may also be aggravated by a fluid intake which is excessive. The mother usually feels sluggish and uncomfortable, with swollen ankles and fingers, the breasts full and heavy, the upper abdominal area tight.

Throughout your pregnancy, keep your salt intake minimal and avoid salted crisps and nuts, or any foods with a high salt content on the labels. Use salt moderately, only in cooking, but not sprinkled on the food itself. If you do need an extra flavouring agent, then try fresh lemon juice.

Where fluid retention is a problem you should also consider taking extra exercise and elevating the legs onto a stool in the evening.

If the problem is severe, you can drain the legs by raising them higher than the body, lying on the bed with your legs resting on the bedroom wall or bed head. This will greatly relieve swollen ankles and legs.

Remedies to consider:

Apis	The area affected is swollen, often tender and sensitive to pressure or touch. All symptoms are worse from heat. Apathy with lack of drive and energy is a feature.
Calcarea	The mother is usually chilly, sweats around the head at night. She may also lack both energy and confidence.
Natrum mur	An important remedy for fluid retention, when accompanied by weakness and nervous anxiety, particularly depression or fear. There is often an unhealthy tendency to avoid other mothers because of tension and insecure feelings.

FOOD CONTAINERS

Care should be taken when china or ceramic plates and cups are used for the preparation of food supplements because of the risk of lead leaching out from lead-containing glazes and into food. This may be a risk when china cups and bowls are used for acid foods such as apple purees and sauces, especially when used as storage containers.

Care should be taken by nursing mothers where other acidic foods and drinks are stored in glazed china pitchers, especially fruit juices and coffee. There may be a far higher risk of lead pollution of food when the china is over 30 years old, because the lead content of glazes in the past was far higher than at present.

Aluminium is a potentially toxic food container (mainly saucepans and pans), which pregnant mothers should avoid using. Again it is mainly the acidic fruits which cause the aluminium to leach out into foods and lead to health problems.

High circulating aluminium levels are believed to cause constipation and irritating skin conditions. There may also be high aluminium levels in tea and for this reason, it should only be taken in moderation throughout pregnancy.

Remedies to consider:

Alumina	Indicated when there has been exposure to high levels of aluminium food, for example from storage containers or a high consumption of tea.
Plumbum met	A remedy when food or drink has been stored in containers which contain lead, for example lead from wine cork seals, lead crystal decanters, certain porcelain containers with a high lead content in the glaze.
Thuja	A useful remedy for adverse reactions to tea drinking.

FORCEPS DELIVERY BABIES

Usually the mother and child are healthy and no additional help is required. But if the labour is unduly delayed or slow, the mother exhausted, or the head is unable to pass through the pelvis, to prevent damage to the mother or the baby, manual assistance using forceps is required.

After forceps, there is usually bruising of the head, or it is deformed following a prolonged period of pressure in the birth canal.

Any distortion or bruising of the head is usually without significance and corrected naturally within a few days.

An episiotomy is routinely performed to facilitate the use of forceps for the delivery. The incision can often be large and painful. Homoeopathy helps to reduce any bruising which may occur and stimulates a quicker healing process.

Remedies to consider:

Arnica	A remedy for the baby when shocked and in distress after a forceps delivery. It can also be of value to the mother when she feels weak, with severe bruised pain, as if she has been kicked in the lower pelvic region.
Helleborus	This remedy is helpful for the baby where the head has been under extreme pressure in the birth canal, with subsequent slow or diminished reactions.
Rhus tox	A remedy for mild irritation of the scalp with redness and tender swelling of the area, irritated by heat, but better for fresh air and movement.

HAEMORRHOIDS

Haemorrhoids or piles are varicose veins of the rectal and anal veins, with grape-like pouching of the weakened venous walls, usually as a result of back-pressure.

The commonest cause is constipation due to lack of dietary fibre, inadequate exercise and pressure from the weight of the uterus on the lower bowel area.

A prolonged 2nd stage of labour, with prolonged pushing because of a difficult delivery, may cause excessive pressure on the venous circulation of the pelvis. In turn this weakens the veins in the lower rectum and anal areas, causing haemorrhoids because of back pressure.

Itchy discomfort often occurs with a slight discharge of mucus. bleeding is frequent because the dilated veins are easily torn causing a usually small amount of bright red blood on the stools.

Remedies to consider:

Aloes	The mother is exhausted with burning sore discomfort in the lower rectum, the piles bleeding. All symptoms are relieved by cold local applications.
Hamamelis	This remedy is recommended when the piles feel both bruised and sore. Bleeding is usually considerable. The discomfort is aggravated by heat.
Pulsatilla	A useful remedy when symptoms are variable. There is a mucus discharge and often bleeding from the piles. The mother has an absence of thirst and symptoms are aggravated by heat.

HEADACHES

These are not usually a major problem during pregnancy unless the blood-pressure is elevated.

In most cases they are minor and short-lasting associated with a migraine, sinus infection, or a cold. If they are severe and persistent, it is wise to see your doctor for a check-up and diagnosis of the underlying cause.

They are often caused by an allergic reaction, e.g. to cheese, wine or chocolate, and sometimes all of these are eaten at the same meal.

Stress, emotional upheaval, or pressure are some of the commonest causes of headache. Pain is typically felt like a constant tight band around the forehead. The headaches are often present throughout the day but eased by rest, relaxation, peace and quiet.

If headaches are persistent, or tend to recur regularly, then this should be discussed with your midwife or doctor.

Remedies to consider:

Glonoine	The head feels heavy and dull, the pain violent, throbbing and worse for heat.
Lycopodium	A remedy for right-sided throbbing headaches, worse in the afternoon and early evening. The pain is often aggravated by delaying or missing a meal, and worse from feeling hungry, for exposure to cold air, but improved if the head is kept uncovered.
Natrum mur	The mother feels exhausted, always cold, with a poor circulation and a hammering headache. She tends to feel worse from heat or sea air, and is better for fresh air or firm cool pressure to the head or temple area.

HEARTBURN

A common pregnancy problem because of excessive acid formation in the stomach, often irritating the oesophageal and gastric lining mucosal areas. This is often caused by repressed (undeclared) anger, irritability or rage, the stomach overactive, hot and sensitive to food or drink. The heartburn is aggravated by alcohol or spicy foods.

There may also be a movement of acid into the oesophagus because of a hiatus hernia, or the size of the uterus in the latter months of pregnancy has displaced the diaphragm and stomach upwards.

The condition is helped by sleeping upright using several pillows and avoiding heavy indigestible fatty meals late in the evening. Always rest after eating and eat slowly, ideally taking small but frequent meals.

If there is an emotional situation within the family, discuss calmly but directly with your partner. Try to deal with any problems of this nature together and always with a minimum of delay.

Remedies to consider:

Argentum nit	A remedy for flatulence with distention and nausea. There is intolerance of heat.
Cantharis	For burning discomfort with nausea or vomiting, worse from caffeine-containing drinks and any pressure on the stomach.
Carbo veg	There is exhaustion with flatulence and distention, relieved by belching.
Lycopodium	Indicated when all symptoms are worse for missing a meal, in the late afternoon or early evening, also from heat.
Ornithogalum	A remedy for severe burning stomach pain with wind which moves from one area to another, nausea or vomiting, and distention of the stomach.
Pulsatilla	Heartburn is variable, with nausea, a dragging down abdominal discomfort which is aggravated by eating rich fatty food or carbohydrate. Thirst is absent. Dramatic emotional mood swings are common.

STRESS INCONTINENCE

This is a common problem for many mothers following a long or difficult birth. In most cases it is the result of pelvic ligament weakness, causing a cystocele or small hernia of part of the bladder downwards through the upper vaginal wall or vault. The hernia displaces the bladder and the urethra, causing muscular weakness and discomfort. The usual symptoms are urgency and inability to hold the urine for long when the bladder is full, with a slight leakage. There is often loss of control and leakage, when she runs, sneezes, coughs or laughs.

It is important for every mother to practice regularly pelvic floor exercises for the first 6 weeks after birth. These are now taught routinely in both ante-natal and post-natal classes. The exercises are invaluable because they help strengthen the pelvic floor muscles and in this way to help prevent or limit the problem.If there are early signs of constant bladder weakness, the exercises should be repeated more frequently, and continued at least until three months after the delivery.

If urinary problems are still evident after this period of more intensive pelvic exercise, the mother should discuss the problem with either her health visitor or doctor. Often, simple physiotherapy treatments are also available, or the mother may be referred to a continence adviser at her local clinic or hospital.

The combination of pelvic exercises, physiotherapy and homoeopathy is usually sufficient to relieve the condition. If the problem does persist and is severe, it may require surgical correction.

Remedies to consider:

Causticum	There is urinary loss from sudden uncontrolled laughter or from movements, also from coughing or sneezing. The urine flow may be erratic, slow or delayed. All symptoms tend to be better for mild damp and humid conditions.
Nux vomica	A remedy for spasms of irritability with bladder weakness or dribbling. Pain or irritation may occur in the urethral region with sometimes blood-stained urine. All symptoms tend to be better for damp conditions and are aggravated by dry cold. Short-fuse irritability is marked.
Sepia	A remedy for dragging down discomfort and incontinence problems. All the symptoms are worse for fatigue, and in the evening when tired. The mother is also worse during cold weather, but is improved by warmth, a hot bath, rest, also from vigorous exercise, such as dancing.

INFERTILITY PROBLEMS

Failure to conceive is one of the most distressing of all female problems and it can be a powerful cause of depression, frustration and marital tension. In all cases, it is important to have a full medical diagnostic consultation and examination in order to ascertain the cause. Full investigation, including a pelvic scan, ultrasonic examinations where indicated and tests of fallopian tube functioning, is usually essential.

The causes are many and often complex. Some of the most common factors include:- scarring of the tubes because of a previous pelvic infection or past surgery in the area, an accident or trauma, hormonal reasons, an actual infection in either partner at the time the woman is trying to conceive, including a chronic bladder infection.

Stress factors are particularly important, related to a life-style that is too hectic, often pressurised and high-profile, with little time to be still or relax and rest. Other factors include sperm incompatibility, a low sperm count, low body weight, anorexia or malnutrition. Recent (1992) research suggests links with smoking, the mothers chances of conceiving reduced by two thirds, to 30%, compared with non-smoking mothers.

Homoeopathy is usually very helpful in these kind of problems and promotes more healthy ovulation as long as there is not a mechanical barrier present in the tubes which requires surgery.

Remedies to consider:

Medorrhinum	For infertility caused by previous pelvic infection. Rheumatic joint discomfort and exhaustion are also a problem. All symptoms are better for sea air and humid conditions.
Mercurius	This remedy is recommended when the woman feels worse at night, especially from heat.
Natrum mur	For long-standing infertility problems, irregular periods, chill and exhaustion. There is often a high dietary salt intake and marked mood changes.
Silicea	The periods are irregular and heavy, circulation sluggish, with cold hands and feet. The woman is underweight and lacks confidence.
Thiosinaminum	For infertility associated with fibrosis or scar tissue, caused by a previous infection or operation.
Tuberculinum	Problems are usually long-standing, the woman thin, exhausted, unable to relax. Her cycle is often early, prolonged, and with a heavy loss.

INSOMNIA

This is sometimes a problem during pregnancy, especially during the latter weeks where the uterus is large and discomfort occurs because of difficulty in finding a suitable sleep position.

Discomfort at night may occur from fluid retention or movements of the baby kicking, also from palpitations or bladder irritation and an urge to urinate.

In some cases the mother is tense and worried, her mind overactive because of worrying about the future and the baby impairing relaxation and sleep.

The mother should try to relax quietly in the evening. It is not recommended to watch highly emotional or dramatic programmes at this time.

Whenever sleep is a problem, the mother should avoid all caffeine-containing beverages, especially tea, coffee and cocoa, because of their stimulant action. Some decaffeinated products may contain up to 10% caffeine and these should also be avoided.

Remedies to consider:

Coffea	A remedy for inability to fall asleep, the mother wide awake, often feeling agitated, tossing and turning. Sweating with gastric burning discomfort is also a feature.
Lycopodium	Recommended for problems of getting off to sleep, often because of worrying about the future, anticipating problems and difficulties. The mother feels exhausted by the early evening.
Natrum mur	This remedy is useful for insomnia associated with anxiety, tension and depression.
Nux vomica	A useful remedy when the sleep problems are associated with indigestion, often with early waking about 3.-4.00 a.m. with morbid depressive thoughts or feeling tense and irritable.
Spigelia	For sleep problems associated with palpitations or stabbing chest discomfort. Exhaustion and feeling chilly are also commonly present.

ITCHY SKIN PROBLEMS

These sometimes occur with a mild eczema around the nipple area which may sometimes become more severe with a clear discharge, dryness and cracking. Calendula cream or lotion can be applied.

The cause is often because the nipple and surrounding areolar area is not kept completely dry after feeding, or where there has been a spontaneous loss of milk, the nipple area damp in the bra, leading to irritation.

Do not use biological washing powders for your bra if they cause any form of irritation and always give a double rinse after use to keep irritating detergent residues minimal.

Always change breast pads as soon as they feel damp. Exposing the breast to warm fresh air twice daily helps healing of an irritated skin area, or exposing an irritated area to warm sunlight for five to ten minutes, also helps to stimulate healing.

If the skin irritation is general, perhaps involving the hands or any other area of the body, the most likely causes is allergy or stress. But always discuss any skin problems with your doctor or health visitor. The response to homoeopathy is usually very positive.

Remedies to consider:

Graphites	For eczematous conditions which ooze a clear or yellow fluid discharge, always worse from heat or covering up the affected skin area.
Rhus tox	Indicated when the skin is thickened, red and irritable, often bleeding where it has been scratched. Most symptoms are improved by warmth and exposure to fresh air.
Silicea	A useful remedy when cracking or infection occurs.
Sulphur	This remedy is of value when there are chronic irritating skin problems. The area is often infected and has a grey discolouration. Irritation is aggravated by contact with water and also from warm humid conditions.

LACTATION, TO INCREASE MILK FLOW

In most cases the causes of the lack of milk is unknown, often associated with insufficient glandular development within the breast. The stimulus for milk production, or 'let down ' reflex comes directly from stimulation of the nipple, sending impulses to the pituitary gland within the mid-brain.

Both lactation and the 'let down' reflex, may be inhibited by tension within the partner, or if the mother herself is insecure, uneasy, or lacking in confidence. When the mother is feeling tense, this is easily conveyed to the baby and may undermine the strength or confidence of sucking. When a baby is weak - does not suck strongly enough - or is unable to properly 'latch onto' the breast, this further weakens the flow of milk.

If the mother is in pain, or has an acute illness, this will also tend to inhibit milk production and should be treated as soon as possible. In other cases the mother is tired, or depressed, reducing the amount of milk production. The more often the baby sucks at the breast, the better is the supply of milk. It is usually recommended to give frequent feeds, i.e. 3 hourly.

To maintain breast-feeding, the mother needs a high daily Calorie intake and a nutritious diet, taking plenty of fluids. A daily intake of up to 3,500 Calories a day has been recommended, but as many women tend to be overweight at this time, an extra 500 Calories a day is often sufficient to meet the extra demands. If she is underweight, an extra 1,000 Calories is recommended during the nursing period.

Remedies to consider:

Agnus cast	This remedy is indicated when the mother is depressed, lacking in vitality and energy.
Asafoetida	The mother is severely preoccupied with her own health. She is very sensitive. The breast tends to throb, especially at night. She usually feels better for fresh air and movement.
Pulsatilla	A remedy when there is a variable flow of milk, the mother often anxious and insecure, frequently tearful with variable mood swings. There is an absence of thirst. Heat in any forms tends to cause an aggravation of her problems and she is quite intolerant of fatty foods.

LOSS OF LIBIDO

It is quite normal for fluctuations in libido to occur, often associated with a particular phase of the female menstrual cycle. Some loss of sexual interest is a very common problem after childbirth.

It is usually psychological in origin, although pain from a stitch abscess or tender vaginal area after a long or difficult birth can also be contributory factors. Anaemia, diabetes, almost any drawn-out physical problem and the contraceptive 'pill' can also reduce the sexual urge.

Excessive tiredness, due to the demands of the baby, night feeds, and adjustment to her new role, also tends to diminish libidinal drive at this time. Breast-feeding can also lead to a lessening of sexual drive and interest, as the mother tends to feel more tired. Some mothers may experience a feeling of sexual pleasure from the baby sucking at the breast, which reduces the need for sexual gratification from their partner.

Fear is often the major barrier, because of pain, or the breakdown of the episiotomy scar after intercourse. The use of a lubricant, such as KY jelly or Calendula cream is a useful aid and source of comfort and confidence at this time.

Discussion of any difficulty without pressure is always helpful, especially where anxiety about intercourse causes tension or anxiety. The open sharing and discussion of fears, combined with holding and gentle stroking, without an immediate direct sexual demand or aim, always helps confidence and relaxation.

Remedies to consider:

Agnus cast	There is lack of sexual interest and drive, often associated with fatigue and depression.
Ammonium carb	Indicated where there is aversion to sexual intercourse, the mother heavy and tired, all symptoms worse for bathing or any contact with water.
Onosmodium	Sexual interest is low or absent. The pelvic and breast areas are uncomfortable.
Pulsatilla	There is a variable lessening of libidinal interest, always worse from heat or stuffy conditions, Mood-swings and tearfulness are characteristic.
Sepia	For sexual indifference with fatigue and exhaustion, worse in the evening, from cold or thunder. An improvement occurs after exercise, such as dancing.
Silicea	Indicated when the woman is thin, often feeling chilly and cold, both libido and vitality are dragged down by recurrent infections, which tend to form a boil or abscess.

MASTITIS

There is an infection of the breast tissue. This may occur following a cracked infected nipple or without an obvious reason. Other causes are obstruction and infection of a milk duct.

Usually a portion of the breast is pink or red, swollen and tender to touch. The mother often has a high temperature with vague flu-like symptoms. She should rest as much as possible.

It is very important for the mother to have immediate prompt treatment for this condition. Any delay, even of 24 hours, may mean that the mastitis gets very much worse and it is important to avoid any complications.

The baby should not be routinely taken off the breast at this time.

The health visitor should always be informed if there is any breast pain, tenderness or swelling.

Remedies to consider:

Belladonna The breast is hard, inflamed, swollen, red and heavy.

Bryonia There is burning pain. The breast feels hot and sensitive to the least pressure or movement.

Cimicifuga This remedy is mainly for left-sided mastitis, the pain worse from cold air or applications.

Hepar sulph For stitch-like pains, the breast hard and tender, discomfort worse from contact with cold air or any pressure.

Mercurius A remedy for a very painful inflamed breast with profuse sweating, the pain worse from heat or when perspiring.

Phytolacca Indicated for right-sided mastitis, the breast extremely sensitive to touch or pressure. All symptoms are worse from humid conditions, and better for local warmth.

Silicea For severe breast infections, usually with a discharge. The mother is thin and weak, always chilly, but preferring damp humid conditions.

THREATENED MISCARRIAGE

Threatened miscarriage is often a recurrent problem, tending to occur at about the twelfth week, although it may occur earlier or later.

There is usually a loss of blood with pain, and either contractions, or colicky discomfort.

The major cause is usually considered to be hormonal in origin, but emotional and stress pressures are frequently a factor, and also infection.

Pre-natal preparation, both physically and psychologically, can help to prevent this condition. Miscarriage is always distressing for the mother and is better avoided where possible.

There are no risks from using homoeopathy at any time during pregnancy.

Remedies to consider:

Arnica	For severe pelvic pains, the area feeling bruised, as if the mother has been kicked. Haemorrhage may occur.
Belladonna	There are severe dragging down pelvic pains, often accompanied by a loss of bright red blood. All symptoms are worse from heat or any sudden jarring movement.
Chamomilla	This is indicated when the pains are severe, with colicky cramping contraction, as if going into labour.
Secale	Indicated when the mother has colicky burning pelvic pain, often with an offensive dark discharge. She usually feels cold and chilled, but is nevertheless worse for heat or if covered up.
Viburnum op	A remedy for severe cramping pelvic discomfort with dragging down pains, usually quite early on in the pregnancy. Weakness or fainting may occur. The mother feels better for contact with fresh air, worse for heat.

MORNING SICKNESS

Morning sickness is thought to be of hormonal origin, caused by imbalance, but psychological factors also play a significant role.

It is common during the early months of pregnancy from the 4th week onwards.

Many women experience morning sickness only briefly, the symptoms mild during the first three months of pregnancy.

But in others it can be severe, vomiting and nausea persisting throughout the pregnancy, causing misery and discomfort.

Before getting up, have a warm drink and also eat a dry or plain biscuit. Eat little and often, as soon as the symptoms of nausea have ended. The mother should relax as much as possible during the day and avoid excessive cooking, also cooking odours (because these tend to aggravate the condition).

Remedies to consider:

Ipecacuanha	There is persistent nausea with profuse salivation and vomiting, always worse for heat or humid conditions.
Kreosotum	The mother feels chilled and very cold, to the extent that the stomach feels ice cold. The abdomen is distended. Nausea is better for heat and warm drinks.
Natrum mur	A remedy when the mother feels cold, exhausted, depressed and tearful, often worse from eating bread, rich foods or fats. She tends to feel persistently hungry despite the vomiting and is often worse from sea air.
Nux vomica	Indicated for persistent nausea, with chronic indigestion, spasms of colicky pain, constipation and short-fuse irritability.
Sepia	A remedy for severe morning-vomiting, with dragging down abdominal discomfort which is exhausting. Irritability is marked, to the point of indifference to others.

SORE NIPPLES

This is often a problem when the baby sucks too hard, or the nipple is not inserted correctly, so that the baby sucks to one side and has not grasped the whole of the areola. It may also happen when the baby is left to suck for prolonged periods when there is an inadequate supply of milk. Most cases start on the third or fourth day after delivery when the full milk flow begins, the areola area of the nipple, engorged and distended, often hard because of the milk within them. The young baby attempts to take the areola into his mouth, but is unable to 'latch on', sliding off the areola. This produces damage, because of too much sucking pressure on the edge or side of the nipple which starts to crack.

It is helpful, if the mother hand-expresses some of the milk, for one to two minutes, to soften the areola. An alternative is a warm flannel on the areola area, which softens the engorged areola ducts, allowing the milk to flow more easily, encouraging correct 'latching' onto the breast. Regular firming, drawing out, and towel-massage of the nipples can sometimes help prevent the problem.

Change breast pads regularly, and expose the sore area to warm fresh air for two half-hour periods daily, morning and evening. Three-hourly breast feeds are best, in this way avoiding the baby staying at the breast for a prolonged period. Frequent feeds, avoid the baby being excessively hungry when put to the breast, when eager sucking would further damage the fragile skin of the nipple area. Calendula cream is a homoeopathic alternative to the more conventional lanolin cream.

Remedies to consider:

Arnica	The nipple feels sore, painful and bruised, very tender to pressure or the slightest touch.
Calendula	This remedy helps to heal a sore nipple which feels sore and full, often painful from the least pressure or sudden movement.
Chamomilla	A remedy when the area is tender and painful, the nipple numb with the discomfort. There are colicky abdominal pains with diarrhoea, together with mood irritability. All symptoms are worse for cold and damp.
Nux vomica	There are spasms of pain in the nipple region, also problems of constipation and severe mood irritability.
Sulphur	The nipple is sore, feels hot, with an irritating discharge. Cracks are common, oozing and often infected. The mother feels worse for contact with water and for heat.

PALPITATIONS

These are common in pregnancy and not usually significant. The exact cause is often not known, but usually considered to be due to hormonal imbalance acting upon the conducting channels of the heart.
They can also be caused by infection and follow a viral flu illness. The symptoms may sometimes persist over a period of weeks or months.

Palpitations are always aggravated by stress, also taking caffeine-containing drinks such as coffee, tea, or cocoa during the pregnancy. Where palpitations are a severe problem, these are best totally avoided.

This condition is often more alarming and frightening than actually dangerous, arousing fears of a possible heart attack. The mother should always rest and relax deeply until the palpitations have ceased, using any relaxation techniques, she has been taught in her ante-natal classes, including yoga or meditation.

If symptoms persist, or are accompanied by weakness or headache, then a medical check-up is recommended.

Remedies to consider:

Aconitum For acute, rapid, full, heart-beats, usually associated with heightened anxiety. Weakness or fainting may be present and a tingling sensation in the finger tips.

Belladonna A remedy for rapid violent palpitations which are loud and sudden, worse from any additional effort or strain and from heat. The beating of the heart is felt throughout the body.

Coffea This remedy is useful for night-time irregular palpitations. The pulse feels full and rapid. Sweating and heartburn are also present. Anxiety is usually present and all symptoms are worse after effort.

Spigelia This is a remedy for a rapid uncontrolled irregular pulse beat causing chest discomfort and worse for effort. Fainting and weakness are often present.

SORE PERINEUM

The perineum or pelvic area is often sore after childbirth, sometimes for several weeks, especially where an episiotomy incision has been necessary.

Bathing with warm saline solution and splashing the area, squatting over a bowl in the bath, is a useful stimulation to healing. Applying Calendula cream to any sore or cut areas is helpful. If the perineum feels bruised, apply Arnica ointment.

Relaxation and rest are essential for about a month after delivery. Rest as much as possible with the legs elevated in a high raised position above the head to encourage drainage and revitalise the pelvic area, but regular gentle exercise is also helpful.

Avoid carrying heavy shopping bags, and if possible, toddlers, as this puts strain on the pelvic floor. As much as possible, avoid all fatigue until the soreness has completely gone.

Remedies to consider:

Arnica	The area feels bruised and sore, worse from movement, pressure, touch or heat, but improved from rest and lying down.
Bellis perennis	A useful remedy for pain in the perineal region, the area bruised and sore, worse from heat and any changes in atmospheric pressure.
Calendula	This is an excellent remedy to support rapid healing of the perineal region after childbirth. It may be taken by mouth, or applied locally as a cream to the sore area.
Staphysagria	A remedy which acts positively on damaged or bruised pelvic tissue. The whole area feels sore and is sensitive when sitting. The mother feels either resentful and angry, or over-sensitive and depressed.

PETS AND PREGNANCY

There are two main areas of pet-related illnesses which may cause illness and affect the baby in pregnancy.

Toxoplasmosis is an important parasitic disease, mainly caused by contact with cat faeces litter, with 800 cases reported in the UK in 1986. In Britain the incidence is about one in 4,000 pregnancies, but in the US, it is as high as one in 200.

The main risk is to the baby, which may have low birth weight and anaemia, with a tendency to bleeding because of a low platelet (clot forming cells) count. In many cases the liver or spleen of the baby is affected and abortion or premature delivery is common. The baby may be born blind, or with a deformed head. Other babies who have the disease, may be born apparently 'normal' but develop eye, brain, or ear disease in later infancy.

Toxoplasmosis is particularly common in the Third World and up to 30% of mothers may be affected with the parasite.

The best treatment is prevention. During pregnancy especial care should be taken after handling any pet, and the mother should always carefully wash her hands after handling even a healthy pet. At this time, pets should be kept out of the kitchen, as they may cause infection to occur. In particular, they should not be allowed contact with any surfaces where food is stored or prepared. Pet food should be kept separate from other household food, with separate containers, and washed separately away from dishes used in the home.

Extra care is needed with a cat litter tray. It should be kept clean and if possible removed and cleaned by another member of the family during the pregnancy, within 24 hours of soiling. If this cannot be organised, thorough hand-washing, or the use of rubber gloves, should be a routine after handling cat trays. The litter should be put into a plastic bag and then put into the dustbin.

Always discourage cats from bringing any prey into the house. Gloves should be worn if the pregnant mother works in the garden, or in soil which may be contaminated with cat excreta. After gardening, wash the hands thoroughly, and also the rubber gloves.

Because of high risks of infection, uncooked meat of any kind should not be eaten, or handled when preparing pet food with raw meat. The mother should not handle or contaminate other food with the juices of raw meat.

If you are pregnant, always wash your hands thoroughly after handling a cat or kitten, and try to avoid or minimise contact with them at this time. Contact with stray unknown cats or kittens should also be avoided.

The Chlamydia organism infects sheep, but it may also affect humans. It is a risk factor during pregnancy if there is close contact with infected ewes, a cause of miscarriage in the wives of shepherds, farmers and herdsmen. About 6 or 7 cases are reported each year, but the incidence may be higher. Care should be taken to avoid contact with lambing or milk ewes that have recently given birth, also with the afterbirth of new-born lambs.

PRECIPITATE BIRTH

This is often due to faulty management of the delivery, usually where the mother loses control of her breathing and pushing. Attending ante-natal classes always help the mother to work better with the midwife to forge a team approach to the delivery. In this way, the different stages of labour can be more easily controlled by both the mother and the midwife.

The main risk is sudden acute pressure upon the child's head within the birth canal.

This may create risks of cerebral haemorrhage, causing neurological damage, or more subtle damage to co-ordination and occasionally to psychological confidence in later life.

The best treatment is always prevention. The midwife should be in close contact with the mother throughout the pregnancy, aware of the overall state of health of the family and any pressures which may be occurring.

If the baby is shocked, in addition to any homoeopathic remedies, it may require oxygen and help in a specialised unit.

Homoeopathy helps to ensure a smooth more regulated delivery.

Remedies to consider:

Aconitum	Indicated within 48 hours of the delivery, when the young baby is shocked, fearful and restless.
Arnica	For bruising and compression in the birth canal, the baby obviously swollen with discolouration, and sensitive to touch in these areas.
Helleborus	Where the child is more quiet, flaccid (low muscular tone), weak or passive. All reactions are slow and depressed, showing a mild shock reaction to the pressures within the birth canal.

PREMATURE BIRTH

Whenever a baby is born early weighing under 5 lbs, it usually needs extra care for a few days or weeks in an intensive care or special premature baby unit. Where the birth weight is over this, the baby can go home and be bottle or breast fed as normal.

Because they are premature, so too are the organs and although fully formed, they are nevertheless more vulnerable to infection or the effects of drugs and may not feed or suck as well as a larger baby.

All premature and underweight babies need careful supervision by the health visitor and regular weighing to ensure that the baby is not losing weight.

The healthy baby should rapidly regain its birth weight and there should be a satisfactory increase in body weight with each test feed.

If the premature baby fails to gain weight as expected, in addition to homoeopathic support, it may require admission together with the mother, into a special unit until the baby is feeding satisfactorily and thriving as it should.

Remedies to consider

Arnica	For reactions of bruised shock, the baby in a weak, quiescent state.
Baryta carb	A useful remedy to stimulate the development of small underweight babies who are slow to thrive or increase in weight.
Silicea	Indicated for the premature baby who remains small and thin, not gaining weight as would usually be expected.

PROLAPSE

The most common problem is mild prolapse of the bladder into the upper vaginal area or vault as a result of strain from a prolonged or difficult labour. The prolapse drags the bladder downwards and may alter the position of the urethra slightly. This leads to leakage or spotting of urine on sneezing or sudden effort. See section on stress incontinence (page 81).

Uterine prolapse may also occur where the vagina drops downwards, from ligament weakness or damage after a prolonged or difficult labour. The usual symptoms are of a dragging down discomfort and fatigue. The condition tends to get worse with age and is aggravated by carrying heavy weights. A ring pessary is sometimes used, but if severe, surgery may be required to re-position the uterus correctly.

The health visitor should be able to advise you on specific exercises to strengthen the pelvic ligaments which support the vagina and uterus and which may improve the condition after a period of several weeks.

Every mother should aim to prevent constipation and the damage which may be caused by straining at stool. She should also aim to keep her stool soft and floating, which is helped by taking a high-fibre (rich in cereal bran) residue diet.

Remedies to consider:

Nux vomica	A useful remedy for spasms of colicky pelvic pain and irritable bladder problems. There is short-fuse mood irritability, worse for dry or chilly cold conditions.
Ruta	This remedy acts to improve pelvic ligament tone, helping to strengthen the pelvic floor region after strain at childbirth. It is often used combined with specific pelvic floor exercises to prevent the condition recurring.
Sepia	Indicated for prolapse which is severe, with heavy dragging down discomfort and pain. Severe irritability of mood and fatigue are also present.

PUERPERAL DEPRESSION

Puerperal depression is a severe form of depression that some women experience in the weeks following the birth. If experienced after the first birth, it is not certain that it will occur after the next. It is much more severe than the common 'blues' which most women experience after the baby is delivered. The condition often begins innocently as a mild flattened state of mood, but quickly becomes more serious and overwhelms the mother. She often feels increasingly useless and a failure, as the depression deepens, developing delusional beliefs which further undermine confidence.

A break with reality develops as an unrealistic state of mind takes over and hallucinations may occur. She may believe that the baby is not hers, has been changed, or is 'against' her in some vague way. In severe cases she may attack or harm the baby, as the normal processes of ambivalence become heightened and distorted by the illness. Fatigue, disinterest, isolation, mistrust and suspicion of others add to the misery and anxiety that is inevitably present. The illness may have occurred before, after an earlier pregnancy, but the mother is usually perfectly well at all other times.

The cause is unknown and there is usually no history of mental illness or anxiety. It occurs in about 5% of women after birth, and is thought to be of hormonal origin, but the causes are still not fully understood. The illness is very distressing for the husband or partner to observe, concerned for the loss of contact and meaningful communication, and for the welfare of the child. Treatment under medical supervision is essential and hospital admission may be required.

Remedies to consider:

Aconitum	A remedy for very acute psychotic states with restlessness, fear and anxiety.
Aurum met	Indicated for the most profound states of depression, often of suicidal intensity.
Belladonna	Indicated for acute delusional states of mind with confused thinking and restlessness.
Hyoscyamus	For extreme states of restlessness, with marked confusional thinking, depression, suspicion and jealousy.
Lachesis	Useful where jealousy and suspicion is marked, with a tendency to become overactive.
Natrum mur	Indicated for delusional states with depression, severe anxiety and tearfulness.
Stramonium	A remedy for delusional states with violence. Hallucinations, states of confusion, and wanting to run away or escape is characteristic. There is also fear of darkness.

PYELITIS

Infection of the kidney is a common cause of a high temperature and loin or back pain during pregnancy.

It may sometimes follow on a bladder infection and is one of the reasons why these should not be neglected.

In many cases the infection is blood-born, and occurs with no previous history of cystitis or bladder problems. The mother is usually very ill and may feel in a collapsed or exhausted state from the pain and high fever.

Any bladder or kidney infection occurring during pregnancy should be treated by a medical doctor.

The mother should always rest as much as possible and ensure that she takes plenty of fluids during the day. Meals should be kept small and light if she has kidney pain or a raised temperature.

Homoeopathic treatment may sometimes have to be combined with antibiotics when it is urgent to have a very rapid response to treatment.

Remedies to consider:

Aconitum	For very acute kidney infections, with severe burning pain, shivering cold and rigors, as the temperature rises. All symptoms are worse from heat or stuffy conditions.
Berberis	An important kidney remedy for burning renal pains, aggravated by standing or walking. The urine is opaque due to the presence of mucus, or it may be blood-stained.
Hepar sulph	This remedy is for stinging, cutting, stitching pains, worse from contact with dry or cold air.
Mercurius	Indicated when the mother feels very ill, is covered with sweat and has a high temperature. The urine is painful to pass, frequently dark and discoloured. She tends to feel worse when lying down, particularly at night. All symptoms are aggravated by warm or humid conditions.

RETURN OF PERIODS

When the mother is breast-feeding, there is often no menstrual cycle until weaning has occurred. some mothers start their period again after a few months at the same time as she is giving the breast.

If the mother is not nursing the baby herself, the periods usually start within two months following the birth, and return to their usual length of cycle.

It is sometimes noticed by the mother, that if a period returns when she is still breast-feeding, that the baby shows some unsettled, fretful behaviour at the breast during the period. This will usually disappear once the period has ended.

If the periods have not returned and no contraceptive precautions have been taken, there is always the possibility of a further, usually unplanned, pregnancy preventing the return of a normal cycle.

If the periods do not return within two months of the birth or after weaning, and the mother is not pregnant again, the following homoeopathic remedies help to stimulate a return to a normal cycle.

Remedies to consider:

Alumina	A remedy for the thin underweight mother with a sluggish circulation and a tendency to constipation.
Baryta carb	Recommended to stimulate ovarian functioning after childbirth. The mother is tired and weak, better for fresh air.
Causticum	The mother is usually underweight, with tearing rheumatic pains of joints or muscles. Catarrh and exhaustion are a feature.
Conium	Weakness is marked, together with anxiety, depression, often palpitations and dizziness.
Dulcamara	Sinus problems of the nose or throat are present, also rheumatic pains, worse for cold and damp. The mother frequently feels chilly because of a poor circulation.
Graphites	The mother feels cold, and is constipated. Skin problems are present as eczema. She is often mildly depressed and tearful.
Pulsatilla	The mother is quickly tired with changeable moods.

PAINFUL INTERCOURSE

This sometimes happens after childbirth because of a very tender vaginal area, particularly after an infected episiotomy incision, or where there has been a stitch abscess.

The use of KY jelly as a lubricant is recommended, in this way encouraging the couple to take a slow, relaxed and easy attitude to any return to intercourse. After the birth, because the mother is often very tired, the male partner may need to arouse her rather more than in the past or during the pregnancy.

Bathing the area with warm, saline-soaks three times daily is often helpful, or apply calendula cream to a tender area.

The woman is often slightly nervous or tense, especially after an episiotomy, in case the wound opens, or she experiences pain during intercourse. She needs care, more time and reassurance from her partner that he will be both gentle and patient.

She may also be concerned about being able to satisfy her partner after the vagina has been stretched and dilated during the birth process. This can be helped by regular pelvic floor exercises to assist a quick return of muscle tone to this area.

Homoeopathy is always very supportive of any anxiety that may be present. It will quickly lessen any pain or bruising that is present.

Remedies to consider:

Arnica	This is a marvellous remedy for pain or bruising after childbirth and should always be used first for this type of problem.
Hepar sulph	This remedy is indicated when there are sharp stitching pains during intercourse, also irritability of mood.
Nux vomica	Discomfort is spasmodic or colicky in type, often associated with constipation and windy indigestion problems. Short-fuse irritability is common, together with intolerance of physical closeness.
Sepia	There is dragging down discomfort, or low backache, with fatigue and exhaustion. Most symptoms are worse in the evening when tired, but improved by vigorous exercise.
Staphysagria	A remedy for sharp stitch-like pains in the vaginal area, with marked discomfort or sensitivity during intercourse. Irritability or haughty critical attitudes towards others is typical, often covering depression and anxiety.

SEXUAL INTERCOURSE

This can be continued throughout the whole of pregnancy unless the woman is spotting or bleeding, when it is best avoided. This is particularly important at the high-risk times for miscarriage - usually around eleven or twenty weeks.

In late pregnancy, when the woman is more limited in her positions and movements by the size of the uterus, it is often more comfortable for a side-position to be adopted during intercourse, but this is best worked out by the individual couple according to what suits them. When intercourse is painful (unusual), this should be discussed with your doctor.

If you are a single parent, with a medical history of raised blood-pressure, because of tensions and pressures, it may be wise to delay a new sexual relationship until after the pregnancy.

In an established marriage or partnership, there is no reason to avoid intercourse where the blood-pressure is raised, unless contraindicated by your doctor. Provided it is enjoyed and not a source of anxiety or tension, then it is likely to help with a blood-pressure problem by relaxing you.

If you don't enjoy intercourse when you are pregnant, or find it unpleasant or painful, always discuss this with your partner and it is then best avoided until you feel more aroused and interested.

Remedies to consider:

Argentum nit	Indicated when the problem is due to underlying phobic anxiety, usually linked to fear of failure and to insecurity. There is great intolerance of heat.
Natrum mur	A remedy for use when the difficulty is related to loss of libidinal interest, linked to underlying depression and anxiety, also with lack of confidence.
Nux vomica	Irritability, tension and spasm, are the major problem symptoms.
Pulsatilla	There is an inability to relax, together with great variability of mood, and a tendency to take flight from closeness, or emotional involvement, due to lack of confidence. Everything tends to be over-dramatised.
Sepia	Depression, indifference and exhaustion with pelvic discomfort are the main features which indicate this remedy. There is a lack of relaxation preventing enjoyment of the sexual act. The woman usually feels better for exercise, especially from dancing.

SKIN PROBLEMS

These are not usually severe during pregnancy. Infected acne spots or boils may occur when there is compulsion to binge on carbohydrates or sweet foods.

Blotchy pigmentation of the face is common due to changes in the melanin pigmentation cells from hormonal causes, similar to the darkening of the areola area around the nipple. This does not usually cause any severe discomfort or problems.

Stretch marks are frequent, especially where there has been a large weight increase and the baby is big. Varicose eczema may sometimes occur with an itchy reddening of the skin over a varicose vein area.

Sometimes the skin feels heavy and solid, over-stretched and uncomfortable because of fluid retention.

If retained fluid is your problem, remember to keep minimal all salt and sodium-containing foods, especially salted nuts and crisps, at this time.

Remedies to consider:

Antimonium crud	The skin is sore, with infected pimples or blisters, often with a thick or sometimes clear discharge. The affected area is worse for contact with cold water or heat. The mother often feels very irritable.
Ferrum phos	A remedy for infected areas of skin, red and sensitive to touch. The mother is pale, nervous and quite exhausted.
Natrum mur	There are dry irritating patches on the skin, especially on the forehead close to the hair line, but also behind the ears, in the warm moist flexure areas of the limbs and on the rest of the body. Small blisters may form, or thickened itchy areas if more severe. The skin tends to be greasy. It is often improved by sun and sea air, but is worse for heat.
Sulphur	The area affected is hot and irritating, usually discharges because of infection, and tends to be persistent. The whole area looks grey and dirty, all symptoms worse for heat and contact with water.

SMOKING

Smoking in pregnancy leads to a small underweight immature baby, with a smaller head and higher than usual (50%) rate of spontaneous abortion.

The umbilical cord is smaller and also the placenta. Because nicotine depresses the respiratory centre of the brain of the foetus, there is reduction in lung and respiratory movement and development.

The risks are reduced if the mother stops by the sixteenth week of pregnancy, but it is far better to stop before the pregnancy, and preferably when it is being planned for.

Passive smoking can be just as harmful for the foetus as for the mother and smoke-filled atmospheres should be avoided. The partner of a pregnant woman should never smoke in the home.

There may be long-term problems for the baby if the mother smokes during pregnancy, with more difficulties during delivery and possible impaired learning and intellectual development.

The effect on learning ability may be long term and still present at the age of ten years. The baby is more prone to infection after birth.

The main risk to the mother at this time, is chest infection and if overweight, an increased incidence of pre-eclampsia, with high blood-pressure, protein in the urine and fluid retention.

Remedies to consider:

Bryonia	Indicated for a dry, irritating, morning smokers cough, often producing small amounts of white or grey sputum.
Tabacum	A homoeopathic specific which helps withdrawal symptoms when stopping smoking. The mother may initially some disagreeable feelings of weakness, chill, nausea, sweating, palpitations and dizziness. The problems are usually aggravated by heat or a stuffy room.

SORE THROAT

This is usually due to an infection or cold and should be treated with homoeopathy at an early date. Contact with influenza sufferers should also be avoided as far as possible.

The mother should keep her general health, vitality and resistance at a high level, by taking a diet which is high in natural vitamins, especially vitamin C and having regular exercise, also resting before she is tired.

The commonest symptoms are pain, difficulty in swallowing, often with a raised temperature and sore or enlarged neck lymph glands.

During pregnancy, if the mother develops a cold, she should not use her voice excessively and also avoid any smoke-filled areas. She should also reduce her own smoking, if this is still continued during the pregnancy. Warm frequent drinks e.g. lemon and honey, help to keep the mouth and throat more comfortable.

Homoeopathy is both effective and safe for this type of problem.

Remedies to consider:

Baryta carb	This remedy is useful when there is marked tender swelling of the lymph glands in the neck region. There is a severe throat infection, the area is red or purple with stitch-like pains on talking and swallowing may be difficult.
Belladonna	The throat is dry and parched, burning hot and red. The mother has a high temperature, is restless, worse for draughts of cold air or sudden movements.
Hepar sulph	Indicated when there are sharp stitch-like throat pains, often with a raised temperature, the area swollen making swallowing difficult. Irritability is marked.
Lachesis	The throat is infected and looks dark red or purple. Most symptoms are left-sided and worse for wearing tight clothing or after rest or sleep.
Mercurius	There is a severe throat infection with a high temperature, the area, red, swollen, and inflamed. The mother is often bathed in sweat, and exhausted. Swallowing is very painful.

SPOTTING AND HAEMORRHAGE

This may be due to an actual or threatened miscarriage. Unless very slight or transient, the mother should rest in bed and call the doctor to see her at home.

In all cases, she should consult the midwife or doctor for an opinion on the necessity for continued bed-rest.

Rest is particularly important if there is a history of a previous miscarriage, or if she is at the eleventh or twenty weeks stage of the pregnancy.

These are common times for loss of the foetus to occur. See also section on threatened miscarriage (page 95).

Continue to take the homoeopathic remedy until all signs of bleeding have ceased completely.

Remedies to consider:

Phosphorus I recommend using this remedy when vaginal spotting is a problem. The mother is often thin and sensitive, easily anxious, flushing up, with a tendency to bleed easily. The mother is always worse from heat, a change of atmospheric conditions, as before a thunder storm. she prefers cool fresh air and enjoys cold drinks.

STITCH ABSCESS

This may occur after an episiotomy wound has become infected and there is redness with local inflammation, often pus formation.

The area may be very painful, making sitting or relaxation difficult. The mother may have a high temperature. Usually the stitch is removed and drainage may be necessary.

The condition must be under medical care and seen regularly by the midwife or health visitor until it has fully cleared.

Warm sea salt baths, three times a day of the area, help to promote healing. Use a bidet to cleanse the area at all other times.

Remedies to consider:

Belladonna	The pelvic area is burning hot and dry, the pain worse from heat or the least jarring or jolting movement.
Hepar Sulph	Indicated for very sharp and painful stitch-like discomfort, worse for cold air draughts or from local pressure, for example lying on the affected area. Irritability is usually a feature.
Pulsatilla	The area is painful, but the symptoms tend to be very variable, rather like the emotions, which swing from positive attitudes to low feelings of tearful despair. All symptoms are worse for heat and better for fresh air and open windows.
Silicea	There is usually a discharge of blood and pus which must be kept drained, the area swollen and painful. The mother feels very cold and chilled, often anxious and lacking confidence.

EMOTIONAL STRESS

The period after childbirth and during the first few months of feeding may be a time of anxiety and stress. The mother is often mildly depressed. She is usually reassured and relieved that the pregnancy is over but feels tired or slightly jaded, at the same time feeling guilty about her feelings. Often she feels trapped by a young baby, out of her routine and in some cases isolated from her routines and friends. Some mothers experience at this time, feelings of ambivalence towards the baby and this may arouse guilt or a sense of failure or depression, feeling she is not like the other mothers. She may feel inadequate to handle and cope with a new and first baby, which worries her, but she may also be reluctant to ask for help or advice.

At this time, the mother often feels a loss of status, especially if she has previously worked, and emotional conflicts are common, often situated around a conflict of interests between home and work. If the mother loses contact with her female support network of friends, she may feel isolated within the house with the baby or child, but drained emotionally. Every young mother needs to create a new network of friends in the home environment who will understand her feelings, and give her help and support when required.

If possible, it is important to discuss fears or worries which exist, before the pregnancy is planned. If not they may become distorted and enlarged at this time. Every mother should try to discuss her fears and problems with her husband or partner as they arise and if they cannot be resolved in this way, to discuss them with her health visitor or doctor.

Remedies to consider:

Argentum nit	Helpful for phobic anxiety problems and panic attacks when there is intolerance of heat.
Arnica	This remedy is of help for stress problems where the mother feels psychologically bruised, exhausted and vulnerable.
Gelsemium	A remedy for anxiety states, with marked symptoms of weakness, often fear of going out of the home and into new situations. Apathy and lack of drive is marked.
Natrum mur	An important remedy for this kind of problem when depression and lack of confidence is a major feature. The mother is usually more tense and nervous with other people, and makes the mistake of isolating herself, which adds to the confidence problems.
Pulsatilla	Indicated when the mother has very variable emotional moods throughout the day, with lack of confidence, tearful depression, low confidence and self-esteem, also intolerance of heat.

TATTOOING, AND THE RISK OF HEPATITIS

Because of the possible risk of liver inflammation with the highly infective and dangerous Hepatitis type B virus which may involve the foetus, it is not advisable to tattoo during pregnancy.

For the same reason, body piercing should also be avoided.

Hepatitis of this type is a serious illness and is best avoided by taking all sensible precautions.

Remedies to consider:

Chelidonium This remedy is indicated for diseased liver conditions, especially when mild jaundice is present, indicating blockage of the bile duct. The stools may at times be pale, or the urine dark, also suggesting a possible duct blockage. There is often pain or discomfort in the liver region, or referred discomfort under the right shoulder blade (scapula). Exhaustion or severe lethargy is usually a feature.

Phosphorus This is another important liver remedy which has the power to stimulate regeneration of damaged liver cells. The mother is usually thin and pale, with an increased tendency to bleeding.

THRUSH

Thrush is due to a Candida or yeast infection. The organism is endemic and present in the atmosphere and in most organs of the body.

The exact reasons for a chronic infection to occur are often unknown, but there is little doubt that one of the factors is a high sugar intake in the diet which encourages the yeast organism to expand in any warm moist area of the body, especially when vitality and resistance are low.

The intake of yeast-containing foods, such as yogurt, or yeast supplements should be reduced and an excess of carbohydrates and sugars should be avoided.

The commonest symptoms are an unpleasant irritating recurring discharge, with redness in the vulval area.

Remedies to consider:

Hepar sulph Indicated when there are sharp vaginal stitch-like pains, with irritation and usually a clear or creamy discharge. The mother is often irritable.

Pulsatilla A remedy for much more variable symptoms, the discharge changeable, often absent for days or weeks, perhaps worse at period times, also aggravated by heat, a fatty meal, and any emotional stress. The mother is easily tearful, often depressed, but her moods tend to vary, almost from one moment to the next. She is always better for fresh air and open windows.

Sulphur This is indicated for more chronic problems, with an offensive persistent discharge, worse for heat and for washing. Windy indigestion and diarrhoea are often present and add to the discomfort.

TIREDNESS

This is very common in the first few months following a birth. It is usually due to the physical demands of the young baby, with interrupted sleep, the fatigue of the delivery, and often a feeding routine which allows the mother only minimal rest. It is frequently also associated with a mild depression and a sense of let-down not easily expressed or shared. The psychological demands at this time are considerable for the couple, but particularly difficult for the new first time mother coping with the needs of her new baby. Everything about the baby has to be planned, thought about, and a decision arrived at. These pressures can be very tiring, but easier once the mother has had the experience of other children. For the new mother, such pressures can cause enormous fatigue during the first few weeks. Discussion of minor worries with the midwife, health visitor, or a female friend with children, is always helpful.

Some periods of rest and relaxation, during the day, away from the baby, is important for every mother following the birth. She should not try to be totally self-sufficient or a 'Super Mum', accepting help from her partner, friends, or relatives. The mother must realise that some aspects of routine, and housework, will have to be left, without worrying about the state of the house, or any disorder. The mother should try to organise some extra help from her partner, sharing the domestic chores. In this way they can both have some time to rest and relax together. She must learn to accept some degree of chaos around her for a few months, and not feel threatened by this. Having a baby, inevitably lead to some changes in the running of the home.

Remedies to consider:

China	The mother is exhausted and apathetic, with variable flu-like symptoms. These are usually worse for touch, pressure, or draughts of cold air.
Kali phos	The mother is thin and pale, with considerable nervous energy, but exhausted and unable to relax. All symptoms are worse at night, when tired and for heat.
Nux moschata	A remedy for fainting and weakness, the mother feels drowsy, moods changeable. She is worse for damp or cold, and feels better for warmth.
Phosphoric acid	Indicated for chronic exhaustion problems, with depression, lack of concentration, diarrhoea and indigestion problems.
Pulsatilla	A remedy for variable tiredness worse for hot stuffy conditions. The mother is tearful, pessimistic and lacking in confidence.
Sepia	For the mother who is exhausted at the end of the day with dragging down pelvic discomfort, often associated with a prolapse.

TRICHOMONAS INFECTION

About 8% of pregnant women develop a vaginal trichomonas infection which may persist after the birth and cause symptoms during the time when they are nursing the baby.

The organism is normally present in relatively small numbers within the vaginal mucosa and produces no symptoms.

But when an infection occurs, the organisms increase in number and cause an irritating and itchy greenish-yellow discharge with a strong fishy odour.

If the bacterial infection is severe, the vagina may become painful, red and ulcerated.

Often both partners need treatment by the homoeopathic approach in order to avoid constant re-infection occurring.

Remedies to consider:

Calendula	This gives relief when applied locally to the area of irritation. It also encourages healing.
Kreosotum	A useful remedy when there is the most intense irritation, aggravated after urination. There is usually a thick creamy yellow discharge. All symptoms are better for exercise and warmth.
Mercurius	The vulval area is red and sore, with a thick greenish discharge, sometimes blood-stained. All symptoms are aggravated when urinating, better for cold water soaks, but aggravated by all forms of heat.
Pulsatilla	There is a creamy or greenish thick mucus discharge, which is variable, worse for heat, better for exercise and fresh air. Mood swings with tearfulness is a feature.
Sulphur	The mother has an offensive thick discharge, the vulval area often infected with pimples or small ulcerated areas, worse for heat, or contact with water.

VAGINAL DISCHARGE

A slight clear mucus vaginal discharge is normal throughout pregnancy, and is without medical significance. The discharge can at times be slightly heavier and more creamy, but provided it causes no persistent irritation and is without odour, it can be safely ignored. At times a vaginitis or local infection may occur, but if in doubt, always discuss this with your doctor or midwife.

Always maintain the highest standards of strict personal hygiene throughout pregnancy. An infection usually causes an irritating, white or creamy discharge, with an unpleasant odour to it which may be of bacterial, viral, or fungal origin.

Vaginal thrush is caused by yeast organisms. These are fed by high levels of sugar intake in the diet, or they may be caused by insulin disturbances as sometimes occurs in diabetes. A high dietary intake is usually associated with sugar craving, eventually causing high sugar levels in the urine, blood, and vaginal mucus secretions, encouraging infection in all of these areas.

If you develop a thrush infection, reduce your intake of sugars and all carbohydrates. Eat a healthy alternative such as an apple when sugars or chocolate are craved. Bacterial vaginitis is also more likely when there are high sugar levels in the diet.

Viral infections are less affected by diet and these should be investigated by your doctor.

Remedies to consider:

Alumina	The discharge is clear, burning and acidic on contact with the skin, worse after menstrual bleeding has ended,improved by cool water soaks to the area.
Antimonium crud	There is a clear watery discharge, which burns on contact with the skin, worse from heat or contact with water.
Graphites	A thin, white or pale yellow irritating discharge is present, The mother is often overweight and chilly, feeling worse during and just after her period.
Hepar sulph	The discharge is thick and offensive. Infection of the vulval region leads to the formation of a boil or abscess. The area is painful, sensitive to pressure.
Lycopodium	There is an acidic discharge, with burning discomfort on the right side of the vagina or ovary.
Pulsatilla	All symptoms are variable with a yellow or green discharge.
Sepia	The mother is exhausted with a thick yellow or green discharge.

VARICOSE VEINS

These are a common pregnancy problem due to back pressure from the weight of the uterus pressing on the pelvic veins and weakening the wall of veins in the area, especially of the legs. Another common cause is constipation where the weight of the faeces in the rectum presses on the pelvic veins and increases back pressure.

Throughout pregnancy it is important to eat foods which are high in fibre, especially cereal bran (preferably organic in origin).

If constipation persists, try to include extra wheat or oat bran in your daily diet until a soft motion is achieved. One or two teaspoonfuls extra of bran is normally adequate to relieve most cases of constipation and to relieve venous back-pressure from this cause.

The pregnant mother should avoid carrying heavy shopping bags or extra weight of any kind and she should rest as often as possible, especially during late pregnancy.

At this time, whenever it is convenient, she can elevate both limbs high above her head, for example when resting on the bed, placing both feet on the head board, or bedroom wall.

Remedies to consider:

Carbo veg	The mother is usually overweight, taking little exercise and lacking energy. She is usually chilly, with a poor circulation, the feet and hands often blue with cold.
Hamamelis	There is a tendency to fluid retention and ankle swelling, especially on a warm day, or in the evening when tired. The feet are often swollen and blue. The veins feel sore and bruised.
Lachesis	A remedy for left-sided varicose vein problems, the lower leg and ankle area has a purple discolouration. All symptoms are worse from wearing tight clothing.
Pulsatilla	There is a tendency to fluid retention and a poor circulation. The mother usually lacks thirst feeling exhausted and weak if too warm, but better for fresh air and gentle exercise. Mood swings are often a problem.

VITAMINS, RISKS DURING PREGNANCY

During early pregnancy there is a danger when Retinol or vitamin A is taken to excess, because it may cause foetal malformation. For this reason, certain foods which are high in vitamin A, especially cod-liver oil, liver, liver patés, and sausages, should be avoided.

Vitamin C is usually regarded as a healthy safe vitamin. There may however be risks if taken to excess, causing infertility, also affecting the cervical mucus and care is needed for women with infertility problems.

Vitamin D in excess may affect the calcium levels of the foetus and overall calcium balance of the mother, causing osteoporosis or bone thinning. For this reason, especial care is needed during pregnancy. You should avoid giving high amounts to young infants, because it may interfere with the normal bone development. Irritability, drowsiness and depression have also been reported, due to its action on the nervous system.

Vitamin E (Tocopherol) in excess may cause raised blood-pressure and cardiac imbalance. It is not recommended for pregnant women who have increased blood-pressure, or a history of it.

Since October 1990, the Department of Health has advised pregnant women, and those expecting to become pregnant, to avoid liver and liver paté, because of high Vitamin A levels. An average (3.5 ounce) portion may contain four to twelve times the recommended daily intake, and could be toxic to the young foetus. Much of the risk occurs in the first twelve weeks of pregnancy.

Remedies to consider:

If there is a health problem during pregnancy, after an excessive intake of a particular vitamin, it is recommended to take the specific vitamin in its homoeopathic potency. This should always be done under medical supervision.

VOMITING

Morning sickness and feelings of nausea may sometimes become severe and persistent from hormonal causes, creating a severe or major problem for the mother throughout pregnancy.

The main risk is from fluid loss or dehydration, but mineral depletion may occur and also extreme fatigue. It is essential that the condition is under medical supervision until it is relieved.

The mother should rest as much as possible and take small plain meals and a high fluid intake, between the vomiting attacks. As much as possible, the mother should try to focus her mind on something other than the immediate problem, encouraging herself to relax whenever she can. Yoga and meditation are very helpful, also the use of acu-pressure bands, available from most pharmacies. These can be safely combined with the homoeopathic approach without fear of undermining its action.

When vomiting is severe or constant, back-up and support will be likely to be needed from the family as the mother is likely to feel depressed, exhausted and debilitated, until the problem is resolved.

Remedies to consider:

Ipecacuanha	There is persistent nausea with salivation. Fainting, watery explosive diarrhoea and twitching of the face may occur. The mother is often irritable.
Nux vomica	Constipation, flatulence, spasms of colicky pain with severe persistent nausea and vomiting is present. Short-fuse irritability, is an indication for this remedy.
Petroleum	Nausea with sweating is marked, with hunger after vomiting. There is dislike of fatty foods, with burning stomach pains, flatulence, and a hollow stomach emptiness.
Sepia	Persistent nausea is present, especially on waking. Weakness, fatigue, with irritability. The mother feels dragged down by her problems and wants to be left alone. She is improved by rest, warmth, and vigorous exercise.
Tabacum	The mother is chilly and covered in a cold sweat, feeling faint with constant nausea, the pulse slow and weak. She feels better for moderate warmth and for fresh air.

WEIGHT INCREASE

Every pregnant woman should endeavour to keep her weight at its optimum level for her age, weight and height and the number of weeks of the pregnancy she is now at.

The mother should avoid all excesses of fluid intake, also of salt and certain carbohydrates, especially the compulsive eating of cakes, biscuits and chocolate.

Note that some carbohydrate, taken in moderation, is of value during pregnancy providing a source of rapid energy, especially when it has a high fibre content.

Exercise is recommended daily to keep weight, circulation, kidney and bowel elimination, body tone, and vitality, at healthy levels.

If there is a weight increase, it is often due to fluid retention, and this should be discussed with your doctor or midwife.

If the mother is feeling anxious, tense, worried or depressed during the pregnancy, she should discuss any problems with her partner rather than trying to deal with them alone or finding comfort from snack-eating between meals. If this is not possible, than discuss any areas of anxiety with your midwife or doctor. It is far better to prevent the problem by sensitive controlled eating during the pregnancy, as losing weight once the pregnancy is over is never easy and can be depressing.

Remedies to consider:

Apis	Fluid retention is the main cause of any weight increase. This is often because of an allergy, especially due to food sensitivity.
Calcarea carb	There is weight increase, the mother is often fair, perspires easily, is always cold, lacking in energy and cold. Anxiety and lack of confidence are common features.
Kali carb	The mother is tired and feeling depressed, with a tendency to wake early at 4-5.00am. She tends to be overweight, cold and always 'run down', with one infection after an other. Sharp, stitch-like pains are present, in the limbs or stomach region.
Lycopodium	The increase in weight is usually due to a craving for sweet foods, especially chocolate.
Natrum mur	Depression is the major factor causing the weight increase, leading to an excessive food intake. A major problem is a tendency to eat far too many salty foods, especially crisps, salted nuts, or to add excessive salt when cooking.

WOUND HEALING, AND SCARS

The healthy mother usually heals quickly and any scar tissue that forms seldom causes problems. The commonest incisions that occur from childbirth are an episiotomy to enlarge the birth canal just before the final stage of labour and from a Caesarian section.

Homoeopathy helps reduce bruising and local pain and to speed post-operative incision recovery. It can also help where scar tissue creates discomfort and also where it is thickened or excessive.

The local application of almond oil will often help to soften the scar and make it more comfortable. It may take several weeks however, before an incision is totally comfortable.

After the birth, it is essential that every mother has a varied wholesome diet, taking plenty of fresh vegetables and fruit, whole grains and if possible, organic wholemeal bread. She may also benefit from a short two-week course of a combined mixed vitamin and mineral supplement.

Remedies to consider:

Arnica	Useful after childbirth, if the pelvic or abdominal area, feels bruised, sore, or tender.
Calendula	This remedy promotes healing and is of enormous value whenever there is a cut or traumatised area.
Hypericum	Of particular value for nerve damage, often with shooting pains, neuralgia, or an inability to relax or rest because of pelvic discomfort.
Staphysagria	A remedy for constrictive, sharp, stitch-like discomfort, also for persistent neuralgic pain. Irritability is often marked.
Thiosinaminum	Indicated for pain and pulling discomfort along an incision or scar. It is also useful for more prolonged scar-tissue problems.

X-RAYS DURING PREGNANCY

Because of the high risks to the young foetus in its early formative weeks, all x-rays should be avoided during the second half of your cycle (after ovulation). This is particularly important if your period is delayed or late, and where there is the possibility of exposure of an early pregnancy to x-rays.

All form of radiography should be approached with care, accepted only on strict medical indications, during the first half of your cycle, and then avoided completely until a new cycle has begun.

This is true for all forms of x-ray diagnosis, including dental and chiropractic films. Throughout pregnancy, x-rays are best avoided, because of the potential risks, unless there is a compelling reason, involving the health of the mother or the foetus.

Ultrasound scans are now increasingly used during pregnancy. At the time of writing, there is no known risk from this type of investigation, but always keep yourself well-informed and do not hesitate to ask your midwife or doctor if the position has changed.

Remedies to consider:

X-ray	Where there is a health problem following exposure to x-rays I recommend using this specific remedy.
Radium brom	This is another major remedy which is useful. for this type of problem, because the energy source of the remedy is similar to x-rays. Chronic low back pain is often a problem, also itchy skin complaints.

INDEX

OTHER INSIGHT PUBLICATIONS

HOMOEOPATHY

Understanding Homoeopathy (£6.95)

The revised second edition of this comprehensive book explains in clear, simple terms the basic principles of homoeopathy, which can be readily understood by the beginner. The author outlines the approach, indications, and choice of remedies for the common health problems of the family.

Talking About Homoeopathy (£4.95)

An invaluable reference book for anyone wishing to understand homoeopathy. The book covers a variety of topics of general interest which offer a deeper understanding and a more challenging awareness of homoeopathy, its indications, potential and scope of action.

The Principles, Art and Practice of Homoeopathy (£6.95)

A book which explains in simple language the principles of homoeopathic practice and prescribing. It includes chapters on :- Dosage, Potency, First and Second Prescriptions, Homoeopathic History Taking and The Consultation. A second section is concerned with Constitutional Prescribing and the role of homoeopathy in the treatment of Cancer.

PSYCHOLOGY

Emotional Health (£5.95)

A unique and major study of the most common emotional problems facing society in the twentieth century. It identifies their causes and symptoms and then explains the best, practical, self-help steps that can be taken to solve them.Simple guidelines are given in order to promote healthier attitudes, changes in specific problem areas, and better psychological perspectives.

Personal Growth and Creativity (£4.95)

A guide to the most effective ways to stimulate and develop personal creativity in order to bring about positive change in creative outlook. The book offers practical guidelines that will lead to constructive results.

RISKS OF MODERN LIVING

The Side-Effects Book (£16.95)

This books describes in detail the most common hazards of our pressurised society, the props used and their risk to health. Chapters include: Developmental Stages of life, Stress and the Home, Sexuality, Over-The-Counter Drugs, Health Products and Vitamins, Medically Prescribed Drugs, Surgical and Cosmetic Procedures, Immunisation, Food and Diet, Social Addictions, Holidays and the Sun, Travel, Sport, Occupations, Animals and Plants, Household Products, Pesticides, Drugs of Dependence and Misuse, Pollution.

Please send s.a.e. for a list of other titles available.